T0316440

THE TRICKSTER
BRAIN

THE TRICKSTER BRAIN

Neuroscience, Evolution, and Narrative

David Williams

LEXINGTON BOOKS
Lanham • Boulder • New York • Toronto • Plymouth, UK

Published by Lexington Books
A wholly owned subsidiary of The Rowman & Littlefield Publishing Group, Inc.
4501 Forbes Boulevard, Suite 200, Lanham, Maryland 20706
www.rowman.com

10 Thornbury Road, Plymouth PL6 7PP, United Kingdom

British Library Cataloguing in Publication Information Available

Library of Congress Cataloging-in-Publication Data
Library of Congress Cataloging-in-Publication Data

Williams, David, 1951–
  The trickster brain : neuroscience, evolution, and narrative / David Williams.
    p. cm.
  Includes bibliographical references and index.
  ISBN 978-0-7391-4397-1 (cloth : alk. paper)—ISBN 978-0-7391-4399-5
(electronic)
  1. Tricksters. 2. Brain—Folklore. 3. Brain—Evolution. 4. Human
evolution. 5. Neurosciences. I. Title.
  GR524.W55 2012
  612.8'2—dc23

                                                    2012007786

To my son Daniel, who when he was seven and
sitting in the back of the car,
suddenly blurted out, "Dad, I've just discovered the
secret meaning of life!"
"What?" I said, having no idea what might be coming.
"There is no secret meaning of life, only life," Daniel said.

Right then and there I knew he was a Buddha, a trickster,
a wise-fool—which he has indeed turned out to be.

CONTENTS

CREDITS

The Signifying Monkey: A Theory of African-American Literary Criticism by Henry Louis Gates Jr. Oxford University Press (1989). By permission of Oxford University Press, Inc.

Permission granted from Burke, T. (ed.). The Infancy Gospel of Thomas (Apocrophy Gospel, 2nd century). De infantia Jesu euangelium Thomae graece, Corpus Christianorum Series Apocryphorum vol. 17. (Turnhout, Brepols, Belgium, 2011).

Permission granted from Hancock Wildlife Foundation for *We-gyet Wanders On: Legends of the Northwest*.

Three poems used with permission from the book *Songs of Love and War* by Sayd Majrouuh and Marjolijn de Jager (Other Press, 2010).

"Ajapa and the Roasted-Peanut Seller," used by permission from The University of Nebraska Press, from the book *Yoruba Trickster Tales* by O. Owomoyela.

"Kwaku Ananse and Aso," used by permission from The University of Wisconsin Press, from the book *African Tales*, compiled by Harold Scheub.

INTRODUCTION

In the Yoruba culture of West Africa, the mythic trickster character, Ajapa, is famous for his musical gifts, through which he can conjure, transfix, and seduce, while bringing much-needed mirth to the world. Like most trickster figures, he breaks taboos, and mocks the pretensions of society as well as the hierarchal structure upon which society is based. He, being a "lowly" animal (a tortoise in this case) still teaches us humans (of which he is also one through the mythical magic that allows such shape-shifting to occur) that we too are animals, who regardless of our trappings of culture still maintain the most basic instincts, the most primal desires.

The trickster is, I believe, a category defined by certain specific traits, that I argue *does exist* in both myth and culture, which for all practical purposes can be called an "archetype." But I am not using the term in a Jungian sense of an archetype emanating from a collective unconscious or some other mystical cause. Rather, this pattern of myths, stories, songs, and personas stem from a universal human brain that is often at odds with itself: hence, *The Trickster Brain*. Trickster attributes occur not only in mythology but also in the behavior of human beings who take on the roles of clown—from the court jesters of medieval Europe to the Heyokas of the Lakota. Sometimes real-life tricksters are seen as sacred, other times profane, but all share characteristics of the mythic tricksters, enlivening in multiple ways the cultures in which they abide. The human trickster, like the mythic one, can be a rapscallion of multiple dimensions or a cultural hero, serving numerous functions in the society in which he or she emerges—sometimes bringing comic relief during times of sorrow; sometimes bringing joyous artistic expression through antics and/or musical gifts; and quite often showing the folly of the elders—giving even the great and mighty their comeuppance. All in all, the mythic tricksters and the human clowns who play them work to turn the social order topsy-turvy, showing all of us how myopic, self-serving, and ridiculous our numerous pretensions are—each of us emperors without clothes.

The fact that the Yoruba trickster figure of myth is also a musician is no accident, as musicians in societies around the world are often tricksters—through musical feats of magic, through musical shape-shifting, through sexual seduction, as well as through their many songs that challenge the status quo. Often, trickster-musicians are shadowy figures who emerge at the margins, crossing boundaries, treading where "respectable" people dare not go. However, in doing so music tricksters are often willing to embrace the Other in ways no one else can or will—not being afraid to shape-shift, borrow, or steal anything—from melodies to tools. They even steal fire from the sun and bring it back for the good of the tribe. And they cross-pollinate, bringing energy and vigor into their cultures. Like emissaries from another realm, tricksters bring us the continually surprising news that no matter where we come from, which continent, which country, which ethnic group or rank, underneath all of our differences we are very much the same.

Soon after learning about the trickster figure in college, it did not take me long to realize that many aspects of Trickster were present in all the artists, poets, and musicians I had both known and studied. Having made a good deal of my living through music since the time I was a teen, I particularly saw strong correlations between the behaviors of musicians and the trickster characters of myth. It dawned on me quite clearly one day that I myself (as a musician, cartoonist, writer) was playing the role of fool/jester/trickster. I began questioning why such similar traits had developed in both the mythic trickster and the musical fools of the world that had been inclined to follow such a contrary path.

Yet, studying Trickster as a graduate student working on American Indian mythology and culture, I was often frustrated. For while I learned about the various trickster incarnations across North and South America, questions regarding the implications of universal patterns were never raised. No one wanted to address the "why" of trickster. That was because the search for universals in literature was deemed an irrelevant exercise in the Humanities, as it was thought that a universal human nature did not exist. But in the current climate of cognitive discovery, and the prominent rise of evolutionary psychology throughout the sciences, the paradigm of natural and sexual selection has infected every area of discourse, even touching departments of literature (though like Issa's poem of the snail—climbing Mt. Fuji—slowly, slowly). Looking at Trickster from a cognitive narrative perspective allowed me to see things anew.

In order to examine literature from a cognitive narrative perspective one must have a basic grounding in neuroscience, evolutionary psychology, physical anthropology, gender studies, DNA research, prehistory, history, world literature, literary criticism, and more. What I have attempted to do in this book is provide such background information from which further analyses of literature from this point of view can be made. Some of the ideas I examine here, like Miller's Ornamental Theory, are still controversial. Many of the ideas I present will be resisted by followers of social constructionism. Yet, I believe that in the end scientific analyses of literature will prevail and the humanities will have to accept the paradigms arising from scientific thought (including neuroscience and biology). Otherwise literary analysis will not be taken seriously and could be relegated to mere superstition.

The premise of this book is that stories are artifacts of the human mind, and as such, should be able to tell us something about ourselves when examined in the context of scientific research on the brain. By prying into the mythology of the trickster figure, by looking at these stories from the perspective of science, I will be making the case that Trickster *should* be seen as a universal human category of literature that emerges cross-culturally because of our biology. Trickster stems from our ancestors, who gave us the genes and brains we carry with us today. Trickster is part of the human story we never grow tired of telling, for the trickster character rises out of a convoluted evolutionary past, making his way continually into the language of our lives because of the ways we are wired.

1

SEARCHING FOR TRICKSTER

The fool is always beginning to live.

—William Shakespeare

Storytelling, universal to all human societies, gives us a way of making sense of the world we occupy and the many contradictory facets of ourselves. Stories are a rich psychological trove of how the human mind establishes boundaries, categories, meaning, intention, and how it deals with conflict. It does this by working through subtle cues of narration, open to a wide range of interpretation. Stories act on us through numerous techniques, such as connotation, association, imagery, metaphor, plot, and motivation of character—playing off the intuitive knowledge we all have about personal interactions due to the fact that we are social animals who must constantly negotiate our way through a world of complicated relationships. In the human arena, we must keep on our toes, judging the intentions of others and making decisions about how to best survive in a world of group dynamics. For while our species has had to confront the perils of an often hostile natural landscape, we have also had to confront each other in endless games of dominance and power as our genes themselves have struggled to survive, reproduce, and make it long enough to create a new generation that will go through the same patterns: learning to walk, talk, sing, fall in love, have children, make a living, and die. And while every story contains culturally specific attributes, untranslatable stories are few and far between. Most stories deal with universal themes we all recognize—the things we value most—love, sexuality, children, dominance, power, the struggle for life, and grief from death. For this reason, we can take stories from both the ancient past and from cultures around the world and feel in sync with them. We understand the problems even the oldest protagonists face. Hence, we recognize Gilgamesh (both the main character and the name given to the oldest intact written human epic) as he begins his quest to reverse mortality and restore his friend Enkidu from death. We understand what it is to struggle against the gods, who at times seem to have created our human tragi-comedy for their own sport, without the slightest concern for the sentient beings they breathed into existence. For the gods send their tsunamis, earthquakes, floods, drought, diseases, and death, while we humans are helpless to confront such terrors, except in the few instances in which we can use our wits to survive.

Since the beginning of time, our survival has depended upon not succumbing to the verities of nature the deities have thrown at us. So we contemporary readers empathize and root for Gilgamesh when he dares confront those more powerful than himself. Rising up against hierarchy we glimpse something of the ancient rebellious spirit in the human character that, while being caught up in the age-old primate/mammal/animal pattern of struggling for dominance and sexual preference, we are constantly in revolt against. What else is a *struggle* for dominance without a desire to topple the powers that be, even as *we* strive for dominance? And while we need society in order to survive, society—with its inherent structures and rules—can be a bane, an oppressive force from which the individual human spirit often wishes liberation. Yet ironically, any particular quest for freedom usually ends with the establishment of a new hierarchical system, a reversal of power that only puts new players into the same old slots. The new players begin acting in the same manner as the old. Hence, new underlings must struggle to become free from new tyrants. If there is one thing we as a species are it is contradictory, all of us con artists in a sense who are also conned. But neuroscience now informs us that instead of the gods having made everything haywire, it is really our brains that are the culprits, fooling us time and again.

According to science, we are the end result of natural selection. We evolved from the same primordial line of ancestry that unites us with all living things. Our bodies and brains developed from older ancestors; we carry the DNA and wiring of those who came before us. The brain itself was never designed, and because of its klunky accumulated evolutionary construction, we are left living in perpetual conflict that religious faith, drugs, meditation, yoga, psychology, and a host of other "treatments" have tried to alleviate. Our brains do not always make us happy or tell us the truth, and one thing we certainly suffer from is bias. We stand where we sit and like to see ourselves at the center of the universe, thinking *our* stories are the ones that matter—our family, our tribe—*we* are what's essential. We're the good guys. Our motives alone are pure. We are like King Lear, when Regan says of him: "he hath ever but slenderly known himself." As individuals, we are usually oblivious to the underlying forces making us do this instead of that. Whether the conflict is deciding which of our children is truthful or deciding which mate might be better, it makes little difference, for we can fall, like Lear, into disastrously wrong choices. And when it comes to romance, we can be as deluded as Romeo, moving out of one relationship into another, believing that this new one is *finally* it: we'll bet our life on it. With war we again are hostage to bias, because ultimately our political decisions are made "with God on *our* side." With faith in our rightness we gladly give up limb and life. Through all of our strutting on this stage few are aware of the actions of genes and hormones as they play upon the psyche: oxytocin, vasopressin, dopamine, testosterone, estrogen, the naturally occurring compounds in the brain and body that are constantly working to affect our moods and behavior, all of which are deeply involved in motivating us to act, wired in us through evolution. Very few of us are aware that evolution has created our brains to think in these particular ways. Hence, we are all fools of one sort or another, as Shakespeare so aptly revealed. The best stories show our folly, exposing our base motivations and hypocrisy.

Stories affect us through emotion and feeling. They work on the subconscious, and they do so because we are wired to understand them. Our brains make and respond to stories. Our minds have developed to think narratively—in parables and metaphors—the language of the brain. Our minds interpret stories before we are consciously aware of having processed them. Our brains have evolved to utilize narrative in relationship to the environment and to other human beings, for survival. Stories, as we will see, have their own stories to tell about how evolution shaped our species. Trickster tales from mythology and the trickster characters from real life testify to natural and sexual selection at work. Mythology from primal people offer us a glimpse into the mindset of our hunter-gatherer relations: the closest we can get to the past 99 percent of human history lived in tribal life. Tribal people, who have been studied by anthropologists over the last two centuries, are the nearest thing we have to traveling back to the Paleolithic mind. Mythic stories are like *living* fossils. Of course, primal people are no longer seen as having brains and thought processes biologically different from ourselves (as was true in the late nineteenth century when Sir John Lubbock wrote of "savage" religions). The notion that all humans basically think alike was championed by Edward Tyler, and this idea has only been strengthened a thousand times over from the discoveries of neuroscience and DNA. But old stories told by primal people *do* reflect primordial themes that are often masked (though not eliminated) in state-level societies and religions. The fact that similar stories occur amongst cultures from all over the globe tells us (just like DNA) that indeed we are one species. But the idea of a universal human nature is still resisted in some circles. The premise of this book is that there *is* a universal human nature, and that similar myths exist worldwide because all humans have evolved similar dispositions.

Science rests on experimentation, the testing of whether a hypothesis is true or not. If evolution predicts, for example, that a transitional fossil of a certain type should appear within geological formations of a certain age, we should be able to go to those sites, dig, and discover if such fossils exist or not. In the same way we might test for a particular fossil in a particular strata of rock, we should also, with a knowledge of human evolution and neuroscience, be able to predict that certain themes might arise in human storytelling, and that mythic stories would reveal something of the way the brain evolved (for in evolution new elements are added on, but nothing is made new from scratch; the old remains). For instance, if neuroscience informs us that that the brain evolved as a hodge-podge, with contradictory modules wired together, we should see evidence of this "dysfunction," of multiple and antithetical impulses, reflected in stories. If natural and sexual selection were important in constructing our brains for survival and reproduction, myths should reflect patterns of thought and behavior that deal with these elements of survival and mate selection. If language and music both derived from courtship behavior, we should see a resonance of such in mythic literature. Likewise, if dominance and hierarchy are wired into the brain (as studies in neuroscience show), we should see such thematic elements in stories across the board. Stories are the mind's way of revealing itself to the larger community and should provide a rich source of insight into our evolutionary past, as well as into the nature of we who are living today, by the very fact that *our brains themselves* are a product of the past. Since we are the contemporary versions of DNA passed down to us from hunter-gatherer relations, we should see evidence of our universal evolution in stories from across many cultures. I am using trickster tales in this quest because they are persistent, ancient, and continue to be told throughout the world. These stories don't go away. They are invented time and again. In the next chapters I will be walking through pre-history, history, anthropology, evolutionary biology, psychology, the humanities, and literature while diving into the new realm of neuroscience. My contention is that the study of literature needs new paradigms built upon scientific foundations in order to be credible. I also claim that by looking at stories through the prism of science we can gain even further insight into the workings of our brain.

2

THE SILVER-TONGUED DEVIL

His heart's his mouth: What his breast forges, that his tongue must vent.

—William Shakespeare

The term "trickster" stems from Daniel Brinton in 1868. Brinton was involved in the collection and interpretation of American Indian folklore. The term for certain characters who exhibit traits of "naughtiness" and "mischief" took hold and was soon used throughout Folklore and Anthropological studies. Hynes and Doty, who wrote one of the seminal books on the trickster character, describe Trickster as a "bricoler," from the French, one who puts together, creates through collage, reinvents and thereby re-entangles the whole mess. Yet, just what Trickster (or a trickster story) is, and how to define him or her, is no easy task, for Trickster is manifested in many disparate forms. He is usually a mythic figure, a god, or god-like deity, who plays endless tricks on humankind. But he can also be the recipient of tricks, initiating laughter with his foils and escapades (in which he often gets the short end of the stick). He can be bad or good, completely greedy and lascivious, or he can become the cultural hero who makes the world livable for human beings. He can even be a messiah, but truth is, he is often savior and fool at once, representing yin and yang embodied in one conflicted being. He or she appears in literature in numerous shapes and forms, manifested often as an animal (everything from spider to turtle to coyote) while simultaneously also being human.

ARCHETYPES

Before we talk about Trickster we need to examine whether such a category deserves to exist. Stories with similar traits are known as "archetypes." The notion that there were universal mythological elements and that all humans shared a "psychic unity" began with the work of Adolf Bastian (1826–1905), who initiated the rise of structuralism as well as Jung's theory of archetypes.

Carl Jung's theory of archetypes was a way of accounting for structural traits in myths he saw reoccurring throughout human populations. Jung tried explaining these universals through multiple theories, one being the hypothesis of an over-soul or collective unconscious—a speculation that was inventive but had no ground in empirical evidence (though Jung himself was very concerned that his explanation for archetypes be scientific). Jung broke with Freud on a number of issues, but like Freud, Jung correctly saw the unconscious mind as the central force in human motivation, and he believed "man's task is to become conscious of the contents that press upward from the unconscious."[1] Jung's archetypes were not set in stone, but fluid, with osmosis occurring between them. According to C. George Boeree, a Jungian archetype is

> an unlearned tendency to experience things in a certain way. The archetype has no form of its own, but it acts as an "organizing principle" on the things we see or do. It works the way that instincts work in Freud's theory: At first, the baby just wants something to eat, without knowing what it wants. It has a rather indefinite yearning, which, nevertheless, can be satisfied by some things and not by others. Later, with experience, the child begins to yearn for something more specific when it is hungry—a bottle, a cookie, a broiled lobster, a slice of New York style pizza. The archetype is like a black hole in space: You only know it's there by how it draws matter and light to itself.[2]

Jung could not find a way to link his definition of archetypes to science and ended up dabbling in every kind of pseudoscience and mystical explanation to account for archetypes, saying that anyone who wants to know the human psyche will learn next to nothing from experimental psychology. He would be better advised to abandon exact Science, put away his scholar's gown, bid farewell to his study, and wander with his human heart through the world. There in the horrors of prisons, lunatic asylums and hospitals, in drab suburban pubs, in brothels and gambling-hells, in the salons of the elegant, the Stock Exchanges, socialist meetings, churches, revivalist gatherings and ecstatic sects, through love and hate, through the experience of passion in every form in his own body, he would reap richer stores of knowledge than text-books a foot thick could give him, and he will know how to doctor the sick with a real knowledge of the human soul.[3]

Fredrick Crews, commenting on Jung's lack of attention to empirical evidence states that there is

no doubt that Jung was himself an esotericist—not just a scholarly student of the alchemical and astrological traditions but a believer in a solar-based life force and in the power of hermetic symbols to reorganize the psyche and even provide a kind of salvation. His collective unconscious and his archetypes, nominally scientific entities, are in fact occult constructs, since no known physical process can explain how the individual can tap into the memory bank of the entire species and summon powers that reside nowhere in particular.[4]

Crews is correct, but Jung's insight into the *existence* of types is still relevant: the causes were just wrong. Sheer speculation without a way of testing a hypothesis leads to bad guesses and superstition.

Joseph Campbell, following in Jung's footsteps, also saw relevance in the existence of mythic archetypes, for Campbell saw myths as fundamental stories that all pointed back to the same underlying source of longing for purpose in the human mind. Campbell believed that all myths were only masks of the deeper, universal primal urge for understanding, implying a universal human nature:

It [mythology] puts you in touch with a plane of reference that goes past your mind and into your very being, into your very gut. The ultimate mystery of being and nonbeing transcends all categories of knowledge and thought. Yet that which transcends all talk is the very essence of your own being, so you're resting on it and you know it. The function of mythological symbols is to give you a sense of "Aha! Yes. I know what it is, it's myself." This is what it's all about, and then you feel a kind of centering, centering, centering all the time. And whatever you do can be discussed in relationship to this ground of truth. Though to talk about it as truth is a little bit deceptive because when we think of truth we think of something that can be conceptualized. It goes past that.[5]

Campbell brought to light a constellation of mythic tales from around the world, and some true insights into their similarities and themes, but even in this quote it is quite apparent that we are dealing with subjective analysis that comes close to mysticism.

Northrop Frye also delved into the archetypical aspects of literature, not limiting himself to mythology but broadening the scope of his work to all literary production. Frye in his attention to universals believed that "what [literary] criticism can do is awaken students to successive levels of awareness of the mythology that lies behind the ideology in which their society indoctrinates them."[6] For Frye, the search for underlying structure was the key point, and from that investigation might emerge undulations of deeper and deeper levels of comprehension. To Frye, this rather undefined and mystical result was also *supposed* to be scientific (though it was not). He believed that the examination of literature should be a "coherent field of study which trains the imagination quite as systematically and efficiently as the Sciences train the reason."[7]

Levi-Strauss developed the field of structuralism in anthropology in an attempt to account for universals, as he also believed that myths allow a look at logical processes that work at the subconscious level. Structuralism focuses on patterns. Structuralism, as the name implies, is a way of seeing things from an architectural perspective. Looking at a roomful of faces in a lecture hall, for example, the lecturer would get an immediate sense of vast differences between people in the audience—individuals with a variety of hair color, eye color, shape, color of skin, differing body types, weight differences, and so on. But if the lecturer could suddenly see the audience through a giant x-ray machine, he or she would quickly find that everyone looked very much the same, so much so that it would be impossible to tell them apart without specific measurements of teeth and bones. Structuralism is such an approach, looking at the skeletal structure of whatever one is observing—a person, a tribe, a collection of pottery, texts, or bones.

Levi-Strauss also wanted very much to keep his study contained within the realm of science, without relying on subjective interpretation; yet there was plenty of subjective interpretation in Levi-Straus's explication of myth: for not everyone will see the same patterns, the same relationships. Critics said structuralism misses the subtle, seeing the skeleton but not the man, and called it just another version of Plato's Forms, hypothetical categories, which move from the particular to greater hierarchal groupings, a search for universals that are themselves mythical in nature. But its demise was unfortunate and premature. Biologist E. O. Wilson believes that structuralism still holds promise for understanding universal principles based upon a Darwinian approach, for that approach is based on the paradigm that *we are biological* creatures at heart, a paradigm that most critics of literature dismissed. E. O. Wilson states that

> the structuralist approach is potentially consistent with the picture of mind and culture emerging from natural sciences and biological anthropology, but it has been weakened by disagreements within the ranks of the structuralists themselves. . . . The [overall] problem [with structuralism is] its lack of a realistic connection to biology and cognitive psychology.[8]

WHERE IS SCIENCE IN THE STUDY OF LITERATURE?

Traditionally, the humanities have been based upon the paradigm of social construction, that humans are "products of arbitrary social conditioning with none but the most gossamer and inconsequential ties to our evolved biology."[9] This viewpoint has saturated the social sciences for decades. It is the belief that culture alone is what shapes us, that we are born tabula rasa, as blank slates. As E. O. Wilson states in *Consilience*, that

> ignorance of the natural sciences by design was a strategy fashioned by the founders, most notably Emile Durkheim, Karl Marx, Franz Boas, and Sigmund Freud . . . [who] aimed to isolate their nascent disciplines from the foundational sciences of biology and psychology. This allowed them to "avoid the roots of human nature."[10]

The founder of American anthropology, Franz Boas, promoted the concept of cultural relativism and trained his students (many of whom became famous themselves: Margaret Mead, Ruth Benedict, Zora Neal Hurston) not to inject personal opinion, cultural, or ethnocentric bias in the study of primal cultures, based on the paradigm of the blank slate and cultural relativism—that all cultures are equal.

There was an anti-empirical and anti-fascist perspective in this stance. Spencer's development of Social Darwinism (taking the biological theory of natural selection and superimposing it onto the cultural, under the moniker "survival of the fittest") was an erroneous misapplication that later resulted in hideous theories and practices, such as Nazi efforts to perfect the race by killing whomever they perceived of as inferior: Jews, gypsies, the handicapped, the mentally ill. While attempting to divorce itself from this perversion, ties to nature and natural selection were cut off when trying to account for any human traits. The followers of Boas took their philosophy of cultural relativity and neglect of biology out into the field, trying to interpret foreign cultures from the blank slate perspective (Yet, some of the ethnographic analysis turned out to be no more than "creative writing," as with Margaret Mead, who in the end saw what she wanted in Samoa regarding sexual behavior, instead of the culture that was actually there). All people were thought to be merely reflections of their cultural upbringing; there was no such thing as a single "human" nature.

UNIVERSAL HUMAN NATURE

A relevant example of cultural relativism can be found toward the end of Hynes's and Doty's book *Mythical Trickster Figures*, where T. O. Beidelman, in his essay, brings up the question of whether there should even be talk of such a cross-cultural "archetypal" character as "trickster," considering the fact that tricksters from one society to another, indeed even within societies, are never exactly the same:

> It may be that Trickster is too general a category and that those . . . who consider characters as culturally disparate as Ture the Spider and Easy Rider may have begun backwards. Unless we know particular Tricksters and their contexts well, we cannot assume that they represent a valid ana-

lytical grouping. . . . What this suggests is that perhaps broad questions of function are unprofitable; instead, we may ask what texts suggest about a particular society's mode of thought and form of organization, rather than raise questions about tricksters in general.[11]

Trying to uncover something of each society's particular mindset and organization is certainly worthwhile, but Biedelman's argument seems akin to saying that if each language is different in its construction of sounds, maybe we should not be talking about "language" in the broad sense, only "languages" that share certain characteristics but which we have no right to group into a single category. But this is ludicrous.

Another reason behind the denial of human nature is because of a political argument that goes like this: if everyone can be lumped together under the rubric of "we're all just human—all the same," then we might as well pave over diversity—that glorious variation of language and culture, men and women: all the variety makes us distinct and unique. It's diversity that counts. In the wake of the bulldozer of contemporary technological and material culture, it is certainly understandable how this conclusion could be reached. And it is true that such ideas as "we're all the same" have at times been used by proponents of economic advancement, whether they be coming from capitalist or communist enterprises, to justify the annihilation of cultures who found themselves on the fringes of "development," outside the big money economies. If we are all just one, then why keep separate from each other? Why protect indigenous people, for instance, who could, and should, be part of the rest of the modern world, the dominant culture: *those people are just "wasting" their time and resources by doing nothing, only worshipping false idols and not contributing to the overall economic engine.* Such arguments were (and often are) used to rationalize brutality and genocide. But there *is great importance* in searching for universals, for as grand as diversity can be— the big downside to our species has always been our tribalism, our awful ability to perceive anyone different from ourselves (in even the slightest way—a shift in dialect, a different body ornamentation, a different god, a different shade of skin) as *less than human*, deserving neither respect or life. As much as it is important to celebrate our differences, that celebration needs to be grounded in our sameness if we are to survive (a prospect that often seems dim, even as our capacity to communicate with each other, to explore each others' narratives, explodes in leaps and bounds).

Believing that there is such a thing as universal humanity is quite different in nature from those arguments used to condone colonialism in the past. As Paul Hogan says, "no racist ever justified the enslavement of Africans or colonial rule in India on the basis of a claim that whites and nonwhites share universal human properties or that their cultures share universal principles."[12]

Cultural relativism led to multiculturalism, but, as E. O. Wilson makes clear, these positions led to the denial of a unified human nature grounded in biology/heredity that placed us in a dangerous place:

> If neither culture nor a hereditary human nature, what unites humanity? The question cannot be just left hanging, for if ethical standards are molded by culture, and cultures are endlessly diverse and equivalent, what disqualifies theocracy, for example, or colonialism? Or child labor, torture, and slavery?[13]

Steven Pinker's book, *The Blank Slate*, is the most thorough and eloquent demolition of the tabula rasa paradigm. He starts with a quotation from John Locke's (1632–1704) *An Essay Concerning Human Understanding*. Locke states: "Whence has it all the materials of reason and knowledge? To this I answer, in one word, from EXPERIENCE." As Pinker notes, Locke, the father of liberal philosophy, "opposed dogmatic justifications for the political status quo . . . touted as self-evident truths," such as those raised by royalty, the aristocracy, the church, and political elites that justified everything from slavery to serfdom.[14] Thereby, the notion of tabula rasa became sacred to liberal thought but at this cost: the denial of a universal human nature shaped by biology.

TEXTUAL AUTHORITY VS. EMPIRICAL EVIDENCE

Yet, in the scientific community nature has recently taken the front seat over nurture, as new techniques have allowed us to see how much genes play in shaping our lives. What emerges is a picture of interdependence between genes and culture, possibly 50/50. Yet, many in the humanities do not want to give up what they perceive as true. The essential problem for the humanities in the scientific age rests upon the question of empirical evidence. The humanities still adhere to social constructivist beliefs, thereby textual analysis often exists without having to pay attention to findings from the scientific community that deal with the non-textual world. Consequently, literary criticism is never required to substantiate claims that stray beyond the text. Thus we have Michel Foucault's ideas that the body and sexuality are cultural constructs rather than natural phenomena, as if sexual selection and natural selection were not the powerful forces biologists know them to be. We have people like Anthony Synnott saying: "In sum, the body has no intrinsic meaning. Populations create their own meanings, and thus their own bodies. But how they create, and then change them, reflects the social body."[15] But to a biologist the bodies of men and women have plenty of meaning and are constantly sending messages that are older than language and much more potent!

Science and the humanities have also traditionally defined "evidence" differently. Renaissance scholars developed museums that were warehouses full of stuff. Every particular thing under the sun was lumped together and housed. However, as Stephen Jay Gould states, the early scientists "rejected such promiscuous ingathering and sought instead to include certain kinds of objects (and to reject others), arranged in an order that would shed light upon the causes and purposes of their natural origins and utilities."[16] Science wanted to find order in the natural world as it looked for universal laws, deciding not to recognize textual authority—the written knowledge of the past. Scientists abandoned texts, looking into nature instead of books: categorizing natural phenomena and creating taxonomy. Texts were revelations from either God or derived from personal inspiration, and neither was dependent upon empirical evidence—thereby faulty. The humanities went with an attention to texts and art, focusing on the culture of Man, through words and images under the premise that *the search for God could only come from His Word as well as through works of art that glorified Him, as we were made in the image of God.* When those in the humanities looked at nature, it was through the prism of art (artificial, not of nature, but above it, *an interpretation of nature*). Art is textual (whether writ on paper, canvas, or marble). Science, on the other hand, concerned itself with "things of the world," with what could be measured, categorized, and pried into.

Even before Darwin, the threat that science was beginning to impose on the culture of art and religion was beginning to be understood. The Renaissance had allowed freedom of inquiry, but with that freedom came disturbing implications regarding the meaning of Man/God/Nature. The rise of Romanticism in the early 1800s was a rejection of the intellectual for the emotional. Romanticism developed the idea of utopian Edenic states full of noble savages living in tune with nature—based, of course, not upon ethnographic study—but on sheer speculation and imagination. This tradition continues in literature departments, where literary fabrications are called fact, even imagined Edenic states, for literary criticism can often be divorced from the tangible world. As an example, Paula Gunn Allen in the following passage insinuates that human warfare has primarily been caused by colonization, and that American Indian peoples flourished in female-controlled tribal units before the European invasion:

> The same forces that devastated the gynarchies of Britain and the Continent also devastated the ancient African civilizations, and we must know that those same materialistic, antispiritual forces are presently engaged in wiping out the same gynarchical values, along with the peoples who adhere to them, in Latin America. I am convinced that those wars were and continue to be about the imposition of patriarchal civilization over the holistic, pacifist, and spirit-based gynarchies they supplant.[17]

While I am equally concerned with the plight of the remaining indigenous peoples, there is no evidence whatsoever to support the gynarchy hypothesis, just as there is no evidence to support the *peaceful past* contention. No society on earth has ever been discovered where women are in complete control or where violence and war are unknown. There is no reason to romanticize native people as noble savages, and matrilineal descent does not equal gynarchy. The creation of past utopias against which the current corrupt world is defined is a specialty of literature departments, for which any kind of free-wheeling poetic interpretation (this has nothing to do with poetry itself) can come into play, since it does not have to jibe with evidence in a world beyond texts. This is where the real crisis occurs: when statements are made that purport to relate truth to non-textual phenomenon. As Gottschall and Wilson state in *The Literary Animal*, "the theories that have dominated literary theory and criticism since the 1960s now only exist in the humanities. . . . [while throughout the rest of academia it is seen that] the dominant theories of human potential in literary studies have been falsified [as a matter of] scientific 'fact.'"[18]

Post-modernists, for example, claim that language itself is nefarious, unstable, and in the end not connected to an exterior world. As such, *everything* can be simultaneously true (though they point out, "truth" usually follows the politically correct dictums of the time). The related claim has been made that criticism is no different than literature—that criticism is just another type of creative writing—but here we're back to semantics—the definition of Art—right? But no. For we have no reliable method to define any word since there are no true underlying meanings. Words really have no referential quality: a post-modernist contention. Anything can be "art." Anything can be anything.

But language, like everything else about us, arose under the constraints of natural and sexual selection to aid us in survival. Yes, science has biases, and everything must be perceived through the prism of individual minds—themselves biased—but in science things *can be proved false*, for science is based upon the idea that experimentation is necessary to validate or falsify a hypotheses, *and every effort is made to prevent bias*. In the humanities, on the other hand, empirical evidence is often not even enough to overturn a critical theory. In this sense, much literary criticism is very much like religion.

HOW DID LANGUAGE BEGIN?

So what about language? Did it evolve in us without having any benefit? Did it not give us any survival value? Is it only a game of interchanging symbols? And is language innately unique to human beings due to some specialized genetic modification or is language part of the continuum of animal communication, as Darwin believed?

The idea of language being innate to our species is nothing new. The Greek historian, Herodotus (484–425 BC) told of a crazy experiment he had been privy to when traveling through Egypt over two thousand years ago, a story which had to do with King Psammetichus:

> The inquisitive monarch, wrote Herodotus, decided to wall up two baby boys in a secluded compound. Whatever came out of the boys' mouths, reasoned the King, would be the root language of our species—the key to all others. Herodotus tells us that eventually the children came up with the Phrygian word for bread, bekos. In addition to demonstrating the

superiority of the Phrygian tongue, the King's inquiry proved that even if left to their own devices, children wouldn't be without language for long. We are born, Herodotus suggested, with the gift of gab.[19]

While, of course, the King was wrong in his summation that Phrygian was the original/superior language (this has to do with our tendency to hear sounds in relationship to our own tongues), nevertheless the legend tells of an ancient intuition that all languages stem from an original that arose spontaneously in Man. We see the same belief of a primal language in the story of Babel from Genesis. Furthermore, for hundreds of years Catholic belief was that the primal tongue was Hebrew. There have been many other languages proposed as the first. In cultures around the world it is often the gods who give the gift of language to humanity. (Universally, everyone tends to think that his or her language or dialect is superior.) There is, however, contained in the Babel story at least the notion of change (though change was initiated by an act from god), and it was the idea of change that eventually led to the idea that languages evolve. It turns out, that instead of having been created and fixed by a deity, languages are in a constant state of flux—more like rivers and streams than rocks: they change like biological evolution, but not toward perfection, not toward a fixed end. What William Jones, an English philologist (1746–1794) discovered can be seen in the following example: the word for father is pitar (Sanskrit); pater (Latin); pater (Greek); padre (Spanish); pere (French); father (English); fadar (Gothic); faðir (Old Norse); vader (German); athir (Old Irish). In each case, a small shift in sound occurred between ways of speaking these words; yet it is clear that some common element between the tongues remain. This realization eventually led to the idea that a mother tongue, a Proto-Indo-European language, once existed for all the descendent languages of Europe, India, and Persia. Languages, it turns out, did not devolve from a god-given perfect tongue—rather every language is continually evolving, meandering and branching off of an older one. Jakob Grimm (from *Grimm's Fairy Tales* fame) took up the task of looking for the rules embedded in these changes, analyzing the ways in which languages shift patterns of speech over time. This led to Grimm's Law. Supernatural explanations to explain the wealth of human languages were now no longer necessary, which followed the abandonment of the supernatural in all areas of scientific inquiry.

Darwin believed language was partly instinctual and partially a learned art, but that it had primarily to do with sexual selection. However, the Darwinian model was officially abandoned in the academic study of linguistics (as incoherently, linguistics sharply veered away from science). Both the Societe de Linguistique of Paris and the London Philological Society (the main conservatories of linguistic research) in the mid-eighteen hundreds decided to ban all inquiries into the formation and evolution of language, seeing it as folly, and that proclamation remained the operating paradigm for over one hundred years.

CHOMSKY

Noam Chomsky, the dominating figure in linguistics throughout the twentieth and into the twenty-first centuries (and often compared to monumental figures such as Darwin and Einstein) also found the study of language origins to be of little interest. Chomsky, counter to Darwin, found language to be completely different from the kinds of communication systems found in other animals; therefore, he believed that only a big language bang in our species could account for the genesis of human language, which was spectacularly like nothing else.

The split that occurred between the physical sciences and the social sciences in the 1950s also has something to do with Chomsky's reluctance to confront origins. The Standard Social Science model, over the twentieth century, defined the disciplines of anthropology, psychology, and sociology. This paradigm was built upon the idea that a chasm occurred between man/animal, culture/nature, and that a different kind of science was needed to deal with each realm: one for culture/man/ language/psychology and one for nature/animals/ biology/physics. The study of linguistics became the methodological basis for the social science platform. Divorced from the "hard" sciences, the social sciences would often veer into areas not regulated by empirical evidence. Examined from this perspective, it is easy to see how the Chomskyian view never had to confront evolutionary theory. It developed in a world where biology didn't matter. But the split is now seen as having been nefarious from the start. As Dylan Evans says, "researchers began to recognize the idea for what it is—the last refuge of the shaky creationist notion of a radical gap between humans and other animals."[20] The contemporary scientific paradigm, known as the Integrated Causal Model, rejects the old assumptions, and in this conception there is the desire for all scientific information to become unified.

Affronts to Chomsky's position in the field of linguistics have existed by such people as Philip Lieberman, who looked for evolutionary causes back in the 1980s, but he and others failed to garner the attention they should have and subsequently failed to topple Chomsky's formidable fortress. With the rise of neuroscience, evolutionary psychology, the explosion of evolutionary theory, and empirical evidence from all scientific research converging, Darwin's view is winning out. With neuroscience, linguists have had to confront the fact that no specific "center" for language has ever been discovered, even though areas such as Broca's are known to affect the production of speech, and Wernicke's the integration of auditory signals. And while it is known that much of language ability tends to be centered in the left side of the brain (through evidence from brain injury patients—who have given neuroscientists the most primary insights into specific functions of different brain areas)—scans of brain activity during the production and processing of language show it overall to be a global phenomenon rather than occurring locally within specific regions. All the theories that challenge Chomsky have this in common: *language has antecedents in older brain mechanisms we share with other animals, which evolved into human language.* There is plenty of evidence that our own particular genius with language was a result of sexual selection, and in the trickster tales we will see how language (the silver tongue) is often employed for the purpose of obtaining intercourse.

SCHEMA THEORY

Schema theory is a model of language development that presents an alternative to Chomsky and also fits well into the current understanding of evolutionary events. Schema theory accounts for language development without the need for a special generator or a one-time invention. In this model, the brain is seen to have evolved a pre-language thought process for story creation (a natural process we share with other animals) through the need to connect cause and effect—a necessary condition for survival of all "higher"-brained creatures. Here, one might think of a leopard needing to put together a story-like strategy to kill a baboon. The leopard has to have some foresight, some ability to project what her actions might entail, and she must be able to choose the best actions, calculating the best chances for her not getting hurt, because a predator is always in danger of suffering a life-threatening wound and must be continually cautious. So, the leopard picks out what seems to be the weakest baboon in the troop. But even then, she could well engender the wrath of other baboons, which is no small matter, for they are powerful animals in their own right, with massive incisors. She might decide for a hit-and-run strategy, wounding a single animal and leaping away to return later after the animal has died and his comrades have left his side. Intelligent animals must put together such pre-language stories that have nothing to do with words. Rather, these develop from an innate process of the subconscious linking actions into a narrative-like account. Like leopards, we humans also employ this kind of a narrative imagery to create stories that utilize neither written words nor sound. For instance, you are at the zoo watching a leopard when you suddenly imagine the animal jumping over the fence and running toward you. Words aren't needed to get that picture into your head. Regardless of the common misconception, you don't need words to think. A silent movie, or a picture book, brings you a story without your needing an internal voice telling you what is going on. In terms of evolution, thought comes before speech in the structure of the brain.

It's easy to see how a basic understanding of cause and effect is necessary for animals that depend upon mental agility to make decisions and act upon them, as opposed to an amoeba, which needs to be able to react and make decisions in a limited sense, but doesn't need to create a story to do so. However, there is something we and the amoeba have in common, which is value. All animals must have some system to regulate good versus bad in order to survive, and it is in the rising complexity of how value is determined that neuro-systems arose and developed. The old disposition system creates instinct). The most base of categories is dual—good or bad, right/wrong, up/down, backwards/forwards. This primary way of dividing the world in two is ancient and of course predates consciousness. This is the value system even a one-celled organism without a brain must have. Yet, humans, for all our cognitive power, also tend to see the world in binary oppositions much of the time (though such a division almost always grossly distorts the complications found in nature and within our social lives). But it is simple, handy, and a binary judgment can be made in the blink of an eye. Sometimes that is all the time we have. In emergencies we must make rapid decisions, and a binary system allows us to make snap judgments (even if we get them wrong). If we get things right most of the time we have a statistical advantage, getting some of our DNA into the future. The primitive disposition (instinct developing) system of the brain deals with elemental binary decision making, while the more recent mapmaking ability of the brain gives "higher" animals like us an advantage, for we can make better predictions and act upon them due to greater information.

As species radiated out over time, the old brain (that still controls the basic life functions) is still there in us, nearly identical to the brains of fish, reptiles, and mammals as we go down the evolutionary line, performing the same tasks they still do in those other species. The brain stem is the old part of the brain necessary for respiration, a beating heart, sexual drive, and for letting us know when we are hungry. As the brain evolved, in mammals for example, it added new areas that allowed for emotional attachment (such as to offspring—children and other family members who share close DNA), as well as new circuitry for greater cognition—for categorizing and making stories. The cortex and neocortex are the newer brain parts, but they are connected to the older parts. In addition, there are two hemispheres, a handy backup system for most animals, in case one side gets damaged, but for higher-level animals like us, the different hemispheres have evolved to do separate things, thereby doubling our brainpower by divvying up tasks. In addition, the brain works in modules (mentioned earlier), which specialize and have differing goals within a single brain.

The pre-language image map/stories of higher-brained animals are the antecedent for language production in humans. The pattern-making ability would have been part of the pre-wiring acquired from the long selectionist process of evolution, which left higher animals with an advanced way of thinking. At the same time, variations on any story theme would be another necessary part of survival, which would necessitate the possibility of altering numerous new neural connections based on experience. Mark Turner argues convincingly in *The Literary Mind* that it was through the development of these small spatial stories (that could be interchanged through the method of parable) that language (and eventually grammar) came into existence. The human mind has the ability to project these parables from one category to another, and from that flexibility, language, as we know it, arose. Here Turner explains:

Consider the image schema *container*. Like all image schemas, it is minimal. It has three parts: an interior, an exterior, and a boundary that separates them. We experience many things as containers: a bottle, a bag, a cup, a car, a mountain valley, rooms, houses, cupboards, boxes, chests, and drawers. Two of our most important containers are our heads and our bodies.

We use the image schema *motion along a path* to recognize locomotion by people, hands reaching out to us, our own hand reaching out, a ball rolling, milk pouring into a cup. . . .

Simple image schemas can combine to form complex image schemas. For example, the *goal of the path* can be the *interior* of a *container*. This combination produces the complex image schema *into*. Alternatively, the *source of the path* can be the *interior* of a *container*, producing the complex image schema *out of*. The *path* can intersect a *container*, producing the complex image schema *through*. Parable often projects image schemas. When the projection carries structure from a "source" we understand to a "target" we want to understand, the projection conforms to a constraint: the result for the target shall not be a conflict of image schemas.

For example, when we map one rich image onto another, the (relevant) image schemas of source and target end up aligned in certain ways. It may seem obvious when we say someone's head is hanging like a wilted flower, or when Auden describes a solitary man weeping on a bench and "Hanging his head down, with his mouth distorted, Helpless and ugly as an embryo chicken," that the verticality schemas in the source images (flower and chicken) and target image (human head) should align. It may seem equally obvious that part-whole relationships in source and target images should align, that a bounded interior should project to a bounded interior, that directionality of gaze should correspond in source and target, that relationships of adjacency should correspond, and so on. But in fact it is not at all obvious, however natural it seems. The specific details of the rich images need not correspond, but the relevant image schemas are lined up.[21]

This ties in well with scientists from Damasio to Edelman, who say that the brain works through pattern recognition and metaphor, as opposed to logic. Patterns in the form of schemas could be overlaid onto each other, creating a nimble capacity for blending.

Similarly, in terms of how the brain evolved, Lynch and Granger postulate that the neocortex itself evolved from the olfactory cortex, which is different from other parts of the brain in that it is associative in nature. Rather than working to map point-to-point information from the environment (which is how visual and auditory signals are processed), associative information has no coordinates. Smell does not require a mapping system showing spatial dimensions. It is the great associative power of the brain that gives us the flexibility for connecting and integrating images and thought so that the constantly shifting parable-metaphor-making nature of language can occur.

It is flexibility rather than specificity that allows human language to encompass such a wide range of ideas, emotions, connotations, and associations. Each word opens up and is linked to other ideas and categories that shift between each other. As Humpty Dumpty said in *Alice In Wonderland*:

> "When I use a word," Humpty Dumpty said in rather a scornful tone, "it means just what I choose it to mean—neither more nor less."
> "The question is," said Alice, "whether you CAN make words mean so many different things."[22]

At the same time, this does not mean that words are utterly nebulous. Without having some reference to the natural world they would have no survival value for our species. The schema theory is elegant in that it follows the dictum of Occam's Razor, which essentially states that "all things being equal, the simplest solution tends to be the best." Lacking any physical evidence of a specific "organ" for language in the brain, lacking any coherent theory of evolutionary development for such an organ, and that it falls in line with other animal thought processes, fitting into selectionist theory, it is a very convincing idea of how we began to create stories and characters, such as Trickster.

But even though language is metaphorical, its evolution in our species offered specific survival benefits because of its referential nature—it was tied to the outer world and to the inner world of the body. It allowed us to communicate ideas like *there is food around the bend,* or *she has a crush on you.* There is much more emerging from neuroscience that hints at how language might have begun from the perspective of the mind-body connection. Antonio Damasio eloquently put to rest the Cartesian split, long a dominant paradigm in Western culture, in Damasio's book *DesCartes' Error* (that mind and body have nothing to do with each other). And the recent discovery of mirror cells (by Giacomo Rizolatti) shows emphatically that the body and brain are connected in profound ways that also align us with other people. When we watch another individual perform an act, the mirror cells in our brains *set off the same activity as if we were performing the action ourselves.* Another similar type of cell, the canonical neurons, fire, according to neuroscientist V. S. Ramachandran,

> during the performance of a specific action such as reaching for a vertical twig or an apple. But the same neuron will also fire at the mere sight of a twig or an apple. In other words, it is as though the abstract property of graspability were being encoded as an intrinsic aspect of the object's visual shape. The distinction between perception and action exists in our ordinary language, but it is one that the brain evidently doesn't always respect.[23]

There is an important link between gesture, a pre-language form of communication, which includes facial expressions (a true universal language for all humans), brain encoding of the outer environment, circuitry linked to motor functions, and mirror cells, whose evolutionary development allowed for much greater social communication. It is from this mix that the human brain likely evolved language, for we see the combination of ideas (like graspability) merging with facial gestures—that could easily lead to mouth formations, and sounds—and desire to communicate, all tied in with social hierarchy, status, and troop relations. Indeed, neuroscientist V. S. Ramachandran is convinced that it was the greater development of mirror neurons (and their linkage to motor functions) in homo sapiens over our ape relations (who also have them) that allowed us to become human beings and for language and culture to evolve.

In Trickster stories, we often see the mind-body connection displayed is surprising ways. Trickster usually thinks with his body. And the body part that controls most of his thinking is his penis. There is no Cartesian split. Trickster tales reveal the physical body's continual needs and desires; in Trickster, Theory of Mind (the ability to ascertain what another is thinking or doing, which mirror cells make possible) is utilized to develop a course of action that will allow him to fulfill his bodily desires. These plans/stories/plots for Trickster usually occur below the level of consciousness. Trickster uses language, music—indeed all the arts—to manipulate so he can relieve his appetites. For him, the number one desire is to mate. Language has a very tangible relationship to making this happen.

3

THE TRICKSTERISH BRAIN

He who joyfully marches to music in rank and file has already earned
my contempt. He has been given a large brain by mistake, since for
him the spinal cord would suffice.

—Albert Einstein

Evolution has left us with brains consisting of various modules that
do different tasks. Some modules are wired together and some are
not. Some modules are conscious and some are not. Modules do not
have to be in agreement, which is why we have the common problem
of wanting to have our cake and eating it too. Some modules want to
know the truth about our circumstances, surroundings, and options,
while other modules work as PR agents for our constructed self and
do not want to suffer truth. For example, studies have shown that
men overall rate themselves as more attractive than do others. But
this modification of the truth actually works to their advantage, for
thinking themselves a better catch gives other modules within the man
greater confidence, and confidence itself is an attribute that plays well
in the mating game. A module not evaluating things correctly, in this
instance, actually gives the entire male organism a better chance of
passing on his genes.

The module theory helps to explain the many perplexities of human contradiction. We can hold opposing beliefs in various modules, which we all do. Some people can go to church on Sunday and act like a total rapscallion the rest of the week, with little care. Surprisingly, there is no "self" in the traditional sense of a little man in our heads pulling levers—the real us. Rather, the whole of the brain works like an orchestra with a conductor who only comes into being once the orchestra starts to play, and all the modules at play make up who we are. It is the global interaction of all parts of the brain that creates self. And the cortex and neocortex that deal with "higher functions," such as logical analysis, are always tied to the older parts of the brain that deal with desires, emotions, and feelings. Instead of being elegantly designed—the most efficient and marvelous epitome of creation—the brain is in many ways a botched construction job leading to endless contradictory impulses as the new and old parts of the brain attempt to work together. Neuroscientist Robert Kurzban states that

> normal brains are like split-brain patients' brains. In a split-brain patient, modules are artificially separated by the surgical procedure and this prevents certain information from moving from one module to another. In normal brains, different modules might or might not be hooked up to one another, and when they're not, information doesn't move from one module to another.
>
> Actually, it's even worse. Because all the different modular systems in the brain are the product of evolution, there is no sense in which connections among modules is the necessary or default state of affairs. . . . So, informational encapsulation—the lack of information flow across modules—is oddly the default. Evolution must act to connect modules, and it will only act to do so if the connection leads to better functioning.[1]

These modules are essentially what I believe the trickster stories give voice to. The human brain, as neuroscientist David J. Linden of John Hopkins says, is

> a cobbled-together mess . . . quirky, inefficient, and bizarre . . . not an optimized, generic problem-solving machine, but rather a weird agglomeration of ad hoc solutions that accumulated throughout millions of years of evolutionary history.[2]

Trickster stories reveal this mess, but they also show how the "mess" is an essential part of our humanity—we wouldn't be *our kind of human* without *these kinds of brains* stemming from *this* evolutionary past. Storytellers around the world have recognized the disparate aspects of ourselves, which has given rise to comedy and tragedy. In trickster stories our many convoluted impulses are not only acknowledged, they are acted out, often in outlandish fashion. This is not to say that the human brain is nothing short of miraculous, a true marvel of the universe, for it is. But it performs in some bizarre and contradictory ways because of its haphazard evolutionary development.

The brain itself consists primarily of neurons (nerve cells), which were discovered in the late 1800s by Ramon Y. Cajal. Neurons have a job to do, which is control what happens in the body, and they must constantly be sending and receiving messages from other neurons in order to regulate and control. Cajal "understood that neurons communicate at contact points called synapses and proposed that synapses can be modified by neural activity."[3] This became known as the Synaptic Plasticity Hypothesis. Building on this, Donald Hebb, in the 1940s, developed what has come to be known as the Hebbian theory:

> When an axon of cell A is near enough to excite cell B and repeatedly or persistently takes part in firing it, some growth process or metabolic change takes place in one or both cells such that A's efficiency, as one of the cells firing B, is increased.[4]

Neurons have, at one end, axons; at the other, dendrites. Neurons usually connect at those points. (Neurons are ancient, coming onto the evolutionary stage at the time that the jellyfish, worms, and snails emerged, and have changed little since). The average amount of synapses per neuron is 5,000, but there can be as many as 200,000 synapses at a neural connection. Electrical signals are passed through the synapses, but very poorly, and there is only a *probability* that information will be passed from one neuron to another through any particular synaptic connection. David Linden makes the point in the *Accidental Mind* that electricity can move through copper wires at the speed of light, but neurons move information like a "leaky water hose," as the axon "uses molecular machines with moving parts (voltage-sensitive ion channels snapping open and closed) to maintain the spike as it travels down its pathway."[5] This is somewhat equivalent to moving barges up and down a canal through locks that must open and close as water levels are raised and lowered. Following the analogy of waterways—where more water flows larger channels are created. Rivers eventually become large enough for boats to move on them, and the bigger the river the bigger the barge that can float. The same is true of synaptic connections. The more they are used, the stronger they become, and the more information is directed down their particular routes.

Gerald Edelman, Nobel Prize–winning biologist, states that the overall basic neural connections we were just talking of, "for any given animal species are selected during evolution and development," which are what create the different "brain areas and cell collections called nuclei."[6] In other words, much of the structure of our brains is pre-set from the evolutionary past, but an equal number of connections occur within the lifetime of an individual as experience itself creates new neural connections based upon what we learn and do. He calls the brain a selectionist system, which is—it turns out—how evolution works overall. Here's an analogy:

Imagine that you have five people living in a tribe who walk into a new land. In that new land is a nasty parasitic predator that can attack and kill anyone, just by touching a person's skin. All five touch this monster, and immediately three people die, but two somehow survive. The only reason the two are left alive is because there was some kind of resistance in their genetic makeup that the others did not have, *beforehand*. The ones left alive had this variation in their bodies since birth, even though they didn't know it; for it had never been called into use before. But the variation was there. They didn't get hit by the parasitic predator *and then create* this genetic protector. It was already a part of what existed in their genome. This is the way evolution works and what "selectionist" means. We don't "learn" new genetic traits; survival depends upon what genetic information is already there at base and how *it* reacts to the environment. Different variations can be called upon when needed, but they were not put in place by anyone's will or design and not created anew by need. What created the variety among the five individuals was random mutation (working within natural and sexual selection). Before these people were even born those mutations had to have occurred in the genes.

Likewise, as we react to the world we live in we don't invent new cells in the brain, but rather we select new pathways from the neurons that already exist, new connections, new rivers, so to speak, which our experiences living in the world make, but at the same time there are pathways already hard-wired into us from our evolutionary past. This makes clear how the nature vs. nurture debate is really a silly one, for obviously our brains become what they are through the influences of both genetic wiring *and* culture. What is silly is when one camp develops an either/or position, defying that the other exists, and overall it is social constructivism that does not want to offer an olive branch to biology and the rest of science, at times calling science just another version of myth.

In conveying information, it always helps to have as many pathways as possible carrying the same, or similar messages—just to make sure the message arrives—especially when you consider that synaptic connections are not very reliable. Here's a simple example: imagine a telephone cable with twenty separate wires all going from point A to point B. The word "hello" is spoken at A and travels to B through ten wires. There's a greater chance that the information will go through if there are ten wires instead of only one. The other ten wires send a message back to A, letting A know that the original message has been received. The returning information is what Edelman calls, "reentry," and may have to do with the fact that we have consciousness of consciousness. "Reentry is the continual signaling from one brain region (or map) to another and back again across massively parallel fibers (axons) that are known to be omnipresent in higher brains."[7] This idea of "reentry" for biological organisms was developed originally by Francisco J. Varela, a biologist and philosopher who used the ancient symbol of the arborous, the snake swallowing its own tale, to relate the necessity of living systems to develop feedback loops that incorporate the environment and the internal workings of the organism, which leads to "the brain writing its own theory, a cell computing its own computer, the observer in the Observed."[8] Going back to my analogy of the telephone lines—of course the brain is spherical, not linear, and the number of synaptic connections are beyond imagination, some 500 trillion, talking to each other. Plus, the brain is constantly processing external data from the senses and merging that with stored memory. Imagine one million billion connections—or as many as all of the elementary particles in the known universe—and you have an idea of the brain's ability to process information to develop both primary and secondary consciousness (as neuroscientist Damasio postulates): a consciousness of self of the body and consciousness of being conscious (which he is convinced began with, and is linked to, the primitive parts of the brain and did not just develop with the neocortex, as is commonly thought).

Evolution always works through adding on, not through wholesale reinvention. Carl Sagan used the example of a city when relating brain development. The city starts with maybe a trading post, then a shanty town, then the new town begins forming around the old town with larger buildings, fancier stores, skyscrapers, until finally we get the development of the suburbs and outlying rural areas. But the essential fact here is that the old town does not go away. P. D. MacLean first came up with this idea of the "triune brain," a brain that still retains the old brain of our evolutionary past. MacLean defined this as the reptilian complex (dealing with basic bodily functions), the limbic system (emotion), and the neocortex (higher thought).

Related to this notion of "various areas of the brain" hooked together, Antonio Damasio (one of the leading neuroscientists in the world) made the startling discovery that there is no process of thought, whether it be logical or metaphorical, involving either memory or response to outside stimuli, that is not intertwined with emotion. He says that we are "feeling machines that think, not thinking machines that feel." In *Descartes' Error*, Damasio asks "are there sociocultural implications to the notion that reason is nowhere pure?"[9] He answers in the affirmative, his overall thesis being that feeling—stemming from emotion and innate ethical structures that we share with other species, is not some kind of pattern of response divorced from "higher thought, but that feeling and emotion are intrinsic to mind and body."[10]

Damasio states that the

lower levels in the neural edifice of reason are the same ones that regulate the processing of emotions and feelings, along with the body functions necessary for an organism's survival. In turn, these lower levels maintain direct and mutual relationships with virtually every bodily organ, thus placing the body directly within the chain of operations that generate the highest reaches of reasoning, decision making, and by extension, social behavior and creativity. Emotion, feeling, and biological regulation all play a role in human reason. The lowly orders of our organism are in the loop of high reason.

It is intriguing to find the shadow of our evolutionary past at the most distinctively human level of mental function, although Charles Darwin prefigured the essence of this finding when he wrote about the indelible stamp of lowly origins which humans bear in their bodily frame. Yet the dependence of high reason on low brain does not turn high reason into low reason. The fact that acting according to an ethical principal requires the participation of simple circuitry in the brain core does not cheapen the ethical principle. The edifice of ethics does not collapse. Morality is not threatened, and in a normal individual the will remains the will. What can change is our view of how biology has contributed to the origin of certain ethical principles arising in a social context, when many individuals with a similar biological disposition interact in specific circumstances.[11]

It is the consensus of neuroscientists that non-conscious interactions among sub-cortical parts of the brain and the cerebral cortex account for 95 percent or more of mental activity, and subconscious mental calculations involving emotion are necessary for survival.[12] When certain stimuli are activated we are wired to respond *through emotion* as part of the brain makes an immediate calculation: danger! "All that is required is that early sensory cortices detect and categorize the key feature or features of a given entity (e.g., animal, object), and that structures such as the amygdala receive signals concerning their conjunctive presence."[13] Primary emotions cause us to act without having to take the time to "think." (Interestingly enough, the etymology of the word [emotion] means "movement out."[14])

The secondary emotional responses are tied directly to the primary: "Nature, with its tinkerish knack for economy, did not select independent mechanisms for expressing primary and secondary emotions. It simply allowed secondary emotions to be expressed by the same channel already prepared to convey primary emotions."[15] But secondary emotional responses run through the conscious, deliberative parts of the brain. So even though our first instinct is to run when we see a bear, the secondary emotional response gives us choices: we can grab a stick, climb a tree, or stay absolutely still and hope the bear will go away. But both primary and secondary responses are emotion-linked.

Feeling and emotion give our species both the impetus for movement and communication as well as the values that we need to make sense of the world of things and the world of social interactions. And whereas some system of value must be wired into all of animal life, in social species who have evolved complex brains and a network of integrated relationships, a system of values becomes an increasingly sophisticated proposition, and "meaning" and "definition" within a group depend heavily upon the evolution of an acute emotional intelligence. With the advent of culture, the intricacies of values and ethics in the form of social contracts, laws, and customs have exponentially increased until we have the incredible array of value systems (codified and not) within which all of us exist, whether we live in a primal society of Amazonia or in the urban cluster of Manhattan. It is value, stemming from feeling and emotion, that makes up so much of what we are primarily concerned with in our daily lives *and through which we primarily use language to address*—judgments of good and bad behavior—*gossip and news*—linked with the more abstract but still emotionally driven areas such as philosophy, religion, art, music, literature, justice, and politics. Stories of "value" are of paramount importance to our species, and trickster stories almost always concern themselves with values and ethics.

4

EVOLUTION

There is grandeur in this view of life, with its several powers, having been originally breathed into a few forms or into one; and that, whilst this planet has gone cycling on according to the fixed law of gravity, from so simple a beginning endless forms most beautiful and most wonderful have been, and are being, evolved.

—Charles Darwin

Every culture on earth has invented stories to account for existence. Hundreds of tales have been created trying to explain the beginning. In one origin story the ancient ancestors crawled out of a hole in the earth; in another the animals came first and one of them was Coyote, who somehow got it into his head to fashion his own feces into human beings. Or the world itself was a giant egg from which we were all hatched. Or we were born from the bodies of whales, or molded from dust, with the breath of God blown into our nostrils. We were created from the imagination of Thought Woman. The Rainbow Serpent rose out of the earth and regurgitated us. Many of the ways people have tried to explain creation have aspects in common—breath, animals, plants, water, floods, sun, moon—the basic elements of the planet we all share and need for survival. But it wasn't until Charles Darwin and

Russell Wallace independently came up with a cohesive theory that explained the radiation of all life from a naturalistic perspective that there was a way to interpret the existence of living things beyond unbridled speculation and fantasy.

There had been intimations of evolution long before Darwin and Wallace—from the medieval concept of the Great Chain of Being (that every living thing exists in a hierarchical relationship to God), to numerous other thinkers from the 1700s and 1800s, such as Lamark (who erroneously believed that evolution depended upon the will of individual creatures to affect their own change, such as a giraffe stretching its neck, which would produce longer-necked babies). The meticulous accumulation of evidence that Darwin (in particular) gathered led to the first comprehensive theoretical framework for understanding both the natural forces and the vast amount of time involved in the process of species transformation.

Darwin had been working on his ideas for twenty years when he received a letter from Alfred Russell Wallace regarding Wallace's similar theory of animal and plant change over time. Darwin and Wallace planned to issue a joint presentation at the Linnaean Society in 1858, but the death of Darwin's infant son made his attendance impossible. In 1859, the book Darwin spent decades researching and revising, *The Origin of Species*, was published. What *The Origin of Species* did was explain how everything alive on earth was related to everything else, that the lineages of plants and animals could be traced through time from earlier to present forms. Darwin's theory stated that these forms had altered, not because they were created by God in new ways, but because these plants and animals had reacted to continual natural forces which had affected the survival of particular individuals, allowing only the most successful in particular environments to live long enough to pass their genes along to a new generation. This Darwin called natural selection. Herbert Spencer, an economist, read Darwin and saw parallels between natural selection and his own economic theories and coined the term "survival of the fittest." But, Darwin himself saw Spencer's term as problematic, for survival can happen for any number of reasons—blind luck, cleverness, specialized ornamentation, and so on—while "fitness" implies brute strength and Machiavellian intent. Many of the subtleties of Darwin's thesis were lost on subsequent theorists, even into this century, but Darwin's and Wallace's idea was one of the world's great watershed moments that called into question every aspect of science, philosophy, and religion, from which we are still reeling today.

Later, in *The Descent of Man, and Selection in Relation to Sex*, Darwin brought out overtly what had been only implied in *The Origin of Species*, that humans (like everything else) were related to previous life forms, and that we derived most directly from a common ancestor to the African apes. Ever since that revelation scientists have been working to refine the details of Darwin's theory in regard to man's descent, while religious leaders have tried either to discount evolution entirely or co-opt it by saying it only further delineates a biblical account that is metaphorical. In the United States, the battle against evolution rages on in rural school districts in Midwestern and Southern states as if we are still in the era of the Scopes trial. But for science there is no controversy surrounding evolution. The theory of natural selection has become the paradigm for all of the natural sciences, continually reinforced by new data and discoveries, from fossils to DNA. Numerous scientists in our century continue to comment upon the profound accuracy of Darwin's observations. For Darwin, without knowing anything of genetics or DNA, nevertheless got most things right. In 150 years of research, not one shred of evidence has overturned Darwin's basic theory.

Recent technological advances have emerged that allow us to look further into nature than Darwin could ever have dreamed of, from DNA into the brain itself—further confirming evolution. Of course, the brain is also a product of evolution, controlled by genes vying to perpetuate themselves throughout the generations while reacting in relationship to their environment. Like every other plant and animal, our brains and bodies have been molded for survival through the long accumulation of genetic material endowed to us by our ancestors. We carry the DNA of the past into the future, while at the same time that DNA makes us who we are now—from the shape of our bodies and faces to the release of hormones that spur us to want to mate with this person instead of that one. Everything from our taste buds to our ideas of beauty has a genetic component. In addition, science has continually reaffirmed that we are indeed animals who evolved here on earth along with every other living thing (we share some 98 percent of our genes with chimpanzees as well as 50 percent of our DNA with bananas!).

The claims once used to prove humans as separate and special have been shown to be specious. Homo sapiens, not long ago, were thought to be the only creatures to make tools, yet we now know that chimpanzees and even birds make tools (crude tools, but tools nevertheless). And where we once assumed that only humans have reason, emotion, and feeling, science has shown that animals cannot only be incredibly smart but they also have feelings like our own. Incredibly, Dr. Lynne U. Sneddon has even shown that fish know pain, which not long ago was an idea most would have thought preposterous.

While Eastern religious traditions, such as Buddhist and Hindu, have always seen animal life as spiritually equal to human, in Western religious traditions the dominant thought has been that only humans have souls (and hence essential value in and of themselves). Animals, though reluctantly admitted at times as capable of emotion and limited intelligence (even in the West), still were thought to be basically creatures of the physical world, not created in the image of god and thereby lacking souls that could outlast their earthly demise. In the West, consciousness has been closely associated with "soul," the implications of consciousness/soul usually swirling around the concepts of mental ability, reason, and self-awareness. No other animal could write sonnets or build pyramids. No other animal could exclaim like Descartes: "I think, therefore I am." Yet, recent scientific evidence points in a far different direction from what Western philosophy has led us to believe. For nothing discovered through science shows us as fundamentally different from the rest of the animal kingdom. We are primates who have evolved in a particular direction that was neither predetermined nor designed. We are animals. Admittedly, we *are* animals who have evolved massive brains, which is why it is so hard for many people today to accept the fact that we could possibly have had an ape ancestry. For those folks, the very idea of evolution defies common sense. For humans can "think," and talk about thinking. Language and thought are often seen as inseparable (though untrue). Language, more than any of our other abilities, seems to propel us light years away from the rest of creation. For language is often seen as the greatest proof of our humanity. But even here, the human/animal divide is collapsing as science has proven over and over again that the forces of natural and sexual selection are the ones at work shaping our bodies and minds. Interestingly enough, in trickster stories the animal part of ourselves is fully acknowledged and humorously provoked—for tribal people were under no illusion that mankind was made in any other way than all other sentient beings and was only different in degree, not kind.

The idea of evolution is surprisingly simple: all life forms change over time due to natural mutations in respect to the environment. In any particular ecosystem, some plants and animals will thrive and some will die. The ones that live long enough to reproduce will get their genetic material passed into the next generation. The environment is always creating pressures on living organisms. A tadpole, for instance, must be able to make it in a certain pond that has a particular temperature and chemical composition. Out of a thousand eggs, only a few will survive—those best suited to that environment. If they live long enough, they will pass on their genes to their offspring. But some ill-suited tadpoles who can't make it in the pond of their birth might be lucky enough to be swept downstream, ending up in a new pond where it is easier for them to live. After many years, if the resultant frogs are separated long enough, different mutations that occur naturally through the replication of DNA will begin accumulating in each group (those from the original pond and those from the new pond)—until enough genetic differences have amassed that the two ponds eventually end up with two species of frog.

The whole of life operates like this. But we see this same pattern as well in culture, which has developed for us humans parallel to the biological world. Memes (the elements of culture) such as words, stories, images, and ideas, like genes, also change over time.

● 5

THE BRAIN OF SEX

I speak two languages-Body and English.

—Mae West

Sex escalated evolution greatly by creating greater chances for change, but it didn't have to be that way. When one tries to imagine a world without sex, it doesn't seem possible. Of all the things we spend our time consumed with, sex is numero Uno. Trickster stories reveal those parts of the brain that still throb below the neocortex, those parts that motivate our sexual desires. But the all-consuming power of lust the trickster stories bear witness to occur alongside the rules and customs of society, alongside culture and its memes. Even such a libertine character as Trickster must operate in a world of constraint. Without restraint, trickster stories could not have emerged. For human cultures everywhere mandate various prescriptions for sexual activity (guaranteeing that an opposing force against restriction would emerge). Even in Puritanical America, one of the most religious countries on earth, every aspect of our media is saturated with sexual imagery—films, TV, magazines, commercials, visual art of every variety, as well as literature: novels, poems, and songs. (Indeed, many have argued that Las Vegas could *only* have emerged in a Puritan country, for repression is the engine for acting out.)

The time and energy devoted to sex for all species is immense. Though we know that the many complications of sex do not make our world any easier, sex certainly makes for an infinitely more interesting place to live in than if we were asexual. Yet, the surprising fact to most people is this: to perpetuate life on earth sex wasn't necessary. As a matter of fact, one of the biggest biological puzzles has been why there is sex at all. Many species propagate perfectly well without it, and being asexual saves a world of energy and stress. From an evolutionary perspective, if it is the selfish genes (as Richard Dawkins brought to light) who are motivating the life force, why would any creature want to split his or her selfish genes with someone else's—in effect halving them? Why not just reproduce in toto? Why not clone? Asexual reproduction is terribly more efficient than sex, and many animals have this ability: bacteria, amoebas, jellyfishes, echinoderms (of which starfish are a variety), corals, tapeworms, as well as some insects, fish, lizards, and frogs. The largest lizard on earth, as a matter of fact, the female Komodo Dragon, can reproduce on her own if no male is in the vicinity. And there are numerous plants that can recreate themselves without sex: they send out runners, or stems, which then form roots of their own. Willow trees do it—dandelions, grasses, sedges, and cattails. Even potatoes do it. In addition many species can reproduce themselves both asexually and sexually, like the Komodo Dragon and like the aphids, who will madly reproduce asexually all summer long, then suddenly have one big bout of sex before the onslaught of winter. Why? If species can successfully clone themselves, wouldn't cloning be the best and most efficient strategy? Well, it turns out that sex does much more than cloning does to make us fit.

SEX, DISEASE, AND COMPETITION

In *The Red Queen*, Matt Ridley deals with the technicalities of sex and genes that most of us have either forgotten from high school biology, or never learned:

Genes are biochemical recipes written in a four-letter alphabet called DNA, recipes for how to make and run a body. A normal human being has two copies of each of 75,000 genes in every cell in his or her body. The total complement of 150,000 human genes is called the "genome," and the genes live on twenty-three pairs of ribbon-like objects called "chromosomes." When a man impregnates a woman, each one of his sperm contains one copy of each gene, 75,000 in all, on twenty-three chromosomes. These are added to the 75,000 single genes on twenty-three chromosomes in the woman's egg to make a complete human embryo with 75,000 pairs of genes and twenty-three pairs of chromosomes.

A few more technical terms are essential, and then we can discard the whole jargon-ridden dictionary of genetics. The first word is "meiosis," which is simply the procedure by which the male selects the genes that will go into a sperm or the female selects the genes that will go into an egg. The man may choose either the 75,000 genes he inherited from his father or the seventy-five thousand he inherited from his mother or, more likely, a mixture. During meiosis something peculiar happens. Each of the twenty-three pairs of chromosomes is laid alongside its opposite number. Chunks of one set are swapped with chunks of the other in a procedure called "recombination." One whole set is then passed on to the offspring to be married with a set from the other parent—a procedure known as "outcrossing."

Sex is recombination plus outcrossing; this mixing of genes is its principal feature. The consequence is that the baby gets a thorough mixture of its four grandparents' genes (because of recombination) and two of its parents' genes (because of outcrossing) . . .

Put this way, sex immediately becomes detached from reproduction. A creature could borrow another's genes at any stage in its life. Indeed, that is exactly what bacteria do. They simply hook up with each other like refueling bombers, pass a few genes through the pipe, and go their separate ways. Reproductions they do later, by splitting in half.

So sex equals genetic mixing. The disagreement comes when you try to understand why genetic mixing is a good idea.[1]

The reason for sex has everything to do with parasites, viruses, germs, and bacteria. Outcrossing is about keeping an individual safe. In evolution, there is always a war going on for survival between animals and those that live upon them. As Ridley states bluntly, "Sex is about disease." Sex allows for new combinations of defense strategies (antibodies) to be constructed through different combinations of DNA. So as viruses and bacteria constantly evolve to invade us, our immune systems are constantly trying to outwit them. Because of disease, asexual species can quickly be wiped out by a single strain of an enemy invader. For they have one strategy, and if it fails, that's the end of their genes. This is why even species that are mostly asexual occasionally indulge in sex. It's an insurance policy. In the same way, sex also creates resistance to the accumulation of bad genes (that accrue through random mutation). Through sex, you are creating not a clone, but an offspring who might have a better chance of fighting off the invaders or the genes that will make you weak. Sex gives an individual a whole new complex of genetic tricks. And it turns out we keep these old genes for making antibodies around for generations and generations, in the event an enemy will pull out a genetic trick of their own from the ancient past and try to invade us with it once again; consequently, we even share (and retain) some of our disease-fighting genes with cows, from way back when we and cows had a common ancestor![2]

DISPLAYS

During mating season, everything from fish to birds to lizards to mammals of every color and stripe become consumed with nothing but sex: they don't eat or sleep, and some don't even make it out alive. It is common for successful bull elk to not live through the winter after a vigorous rut, the strain of mating and rounding up a harem of cows depleting every ounce of the bull's strength (but still: his genes survive). For females too, the courtship rituals are often intense and consuming. For females the act of laying eggs or going through pregnancy presents great difficulties, which can rob them of energy or cost them their lives.

But the one biological fact that determines the differences in how males and females behave comes from the great disparity in the distribution of sexual cells. In humans, for example, the female has one egg at a time that may be fertilized, while a man produces 250 to 500 million sperm for every ejaculate. This is the reason that, throughout most of the animal world, the female must be pursued. She has more at stake in the mating process and has to be extremely picky. In the animal world it is the female who chooses her partner. She has only one vehicle for passing on her genes: her single or handful of eggs. Nature has programmed females to desire the best genes for their offspring, which means they are attracted to the most successful males, those who portray dominance and virility.

In many bird species monogamous behavior occurs because of the necessity of both males and females hatching the eggs and raising chicks. In order to incubate, one parent must sit on the eggs at all times while the other goes off and procures food. If the female picks a mate who is a deadbeat, who is negligent in his duties, her chicks won't survive. But the loyal mate may not always be the sexiest one on the block. Males and females have different sexual strategies because of their reproductive anatomy. Theoretically, a male can impregnate an endless number of females. In the case of the most handsome male birds (whose bright colors equal fitness)—they will be highly sought after by females—but it is in the interest of these pretty-boy males to inseminate as many of these star-struck females as possible (for they will have more offspring)—letting some other drabber looking male falsely believe that he is the father. Surprisingly, DNA studies have confirmed that even in bird species thought previously to be monogamous, nearly 40 percent of females cheat. She can have her cake and eat it too if she sneaks off with the flashy male, and *doesn't get caught* by her boring "husband." But if the drabber husband discovers that he's been cuckolded, he's out, and the female will have no one to help her sit on the eggs or raise her chicks when they hatch. The good-looking player who really mated with her is already far down the road, no doubt having a dalliance with another gal bird looking for some flash. (It turns out that in birds, the best-looking males are often not loyal.) An entire mating season will have occurred without propagation of a single life. It's all a very risky game in which the stakes are enormously high. Sex goes far beyond men are from Mars and women are from Venus. It's a Herculean life and death struggle, and the entire survival of the species depends upon sexual success.

What leads to the physical differences between males and females is polygyny—a male with multiple female breeding partners, (though Darwin showed that even in monogamous relationships change can occur between males and females, more slowly, through the fact that the offspring of "fitter" parents will be much more likely to survive and pass on their genes). The flashier males have more offspring because the females desire them, and the males have more sexual partners and more chicks. The next generation of males tends to have more outlandish feathers because of this. Females also get the genes for desiring these kinds of flashy feathers over the ones without pizzazz. The process of excessive traits developing, like the iridescent feathers of many male birds, is called the Runaway Theory, developed in the 1930s by R. A. Fisher. Through transference, to *both males and females*, the next generation will have flashier feathers. Males want sex and will get it wherever they can, so there's no pressure on them to be picky. Even if they have a special mate, it doesn't matter. If they can get a little action on the side, they'll go for it, as it only adds to their genetic legacy. The thing is, the male doesn't care one whit if a female looks flashy or drab. For him, a female's a female. But the picky females will *only go* after the flash (for the flash indicates fitness), so once these preferences and mating practices come into play over generations we get what we see in nature: males with fantastic plumage and females who often look dull by comparison. But males and females can lie. From the genes' perspective, the point is to reproduce. What looks good on the male doesn't have to really be good so long as it attracts a mate. The female needs to make reliable decisions based on truth, not deception. The health of her eggs depends upon it. So the male must show that he's the real deal and be able to beat off the pretenders through some method. Darwin, before coming up with the solution of sexual selection to explain exaggerated forms in nature, was very worried that extreme markers would contradict everything about natural selection. A woolly mammoth with tusks too big to carry around would not be good for much. The peacock's tail drove Darwin insane. But he finally figured it out. Sexual selection is the process by which (primarily) females choose males, and this choosing has led to nearly all the marvels of color and design we see in the animal kingdom, from feathers and scales to the cuttlefish's electronic skin.

In 1997 A. Zahavi brought out the Handicap Principal, which further explained why extremism could still benefit a species. When a male takes on the burden of extra baggage it represents additional strength and vitality to carry the extra "weight." In other words, males in some species evolved ridiculous burdens to prove they were not faking it. To carry huge tails, antlers, or tusks is not an easy thing to do; as a matter of fact it's often quite dangerous. A Bird of Paradise can't easily fly from a jaguar; a bull elk can get his antlers tangled in a tree or hooked up with another male and die. These things happen in nature. But even though these sexually selected traits might seem "foolhardy" to us, what they prove to the females is that this guy must be *really macho* to be able to handle all that extra baggage. He is super-fit.

When extremism is found in nature, from the throbbing hues of tropical fish, to the massive antlers of moose, it's a sign that sexual selection has been at work. Handicap traits might show that an animal is extra healthy, free of parasites and disease. Of course, there will always be physical constraints against how far the Handicap Principal can go, which probably explains why many species, such as the Irish elk, went extinct. If antlers get too big for the males to carry successfully, the males (and species) will die. Extinction has happened tens of thousand of times in the past as a matter of fact most animals that ever lived have gone extinct. But regardless of the danger of the Handicap Principal, sexual selection has given us the great raft of diversity we see today—the fantastic radiation of life in its myriad forms—and possibly the very best things about our own species.

It seems strange to us that in most other species it is the male who is adorned with the brightest feathers or most extreme projections, such as antlers, while in humans it seems to be the females of our species who have more "eye candy." But we humans have also developed culture, and in most primal cultures the fashion and rank displays, such as feathered headdresses, piercings, body paint, tattoos, and other adornments are utilized by men as status symbols of wealth and power. In the modern world, status symbols, such as Porsches and Mercedes Benzes, also tend to be most often associated with male displays of hierarchy. But the human animal is also quite different in two ways from other primates—1). In our species, *both males and females are involved in intense competition for mates.* In birds, the male is always ready for a dalliance. But in humans, the survival of one's DNA depends on a much more concentrated and lengthy process of cooperation, as a human child takes well over a decade to raise. Those children that had both a mother and a father around to provide resources and parenting (as well as a grandma) had a greater chance of survival than those who had a mother alone. As a consequence of this sexual competition, both males and females have an intense interest in displays for fitness (still, more for males); consequently, females *also* show specialized physical attractors, such as pronounced breasts and more juvenile faces. Because so much is at stake in terms of a child living to adulthood, females will fight vigorously for their mate in order not to lose out on valuable resources the husband can provide. These emotions are manifested as love and attachment. Jealousy evolved as a radar system to detect signs of cheating and to fuel rage at threatening behavior from a spouse. The male can also become extremely jealous and protective of his mate. The "double standard" arises from the fact that the male still desires to spread his genes throughout the population, which can often be done in secret, with paternity never being able to be detected in ancient times; but for the female there is no hiding the fact that her child is hers, while the male desires a guarantee of fidelity. It is to the advantage of his DNA that no other male be allowed to mate with his female. The energy he puts into parenting does no good to his DNA legacy if he unwittingly raises another male's offspring.

Another thing that makes males and females different in our species is our separate work roles (rare in nature), which evolved as hunting/gathering and do not occur in other primates yet are seen in nearly all primal human societies. Because of separate specialized work, males and females have evolved in some unique ways regarding socialization, communication, and brain specialization, even though overall intelligence for both is the same.

Without sex, we wouldn't have the great variety of creatures that exist today, and many species would long ago have perished. And since sex is so important, much of what we do—everything from putting on makeup, to indulging in bar talk, to buying flowers, to making sure our hair is groomed, or that we've bought tickets to the play, all boil down at the evolutionary level to finding the best genes to insure our offspring will survive. But that doesn't mean we have to be conscious of our motives (natural and sexual selection demand that we do not). So usually we're oblivious as to why we do this instead of that. Most of what we "think" is through the subconscious anyway, some 95 percent. No teenager is dreaming of fighting potential parasites for their future young when they're in a car somewhere having sex. But if we are engaging in all of this sexual activity in order be the fittest survivors in the game of natural selection, just who are we actually competing against? The answer to that question was originally asked and answered by Nicholas

Humphrey. He said, "Selection within the species is always going to be more important than selection between the species."[3]

We are competing against other human beings for the continuation of our genes—not lions and tigers: what counts in this race is who *within the population of our species* will be most successful in spreading his or her genes into the future. As David Buss, in *The Evolution of Desire* states, it was Darwin who first stated that sexual selection takes two forms:

> In one form, members of the same sex compete with each other, and the outcome of their contest gives the winner greater sexual access to members of the opposite sex. Two stags locking horns in combat is the prototypical image of this intrasexual competition. The characteristics that lead to success in contests of this kind, such as greater strength, intelligence, or attractiveness to allies, evolve because the victors are able to mate more often and hence pass on more genes. In the other type of sexual selection, members of one sex choose a mate based on their preferences for particular qualities in that mate.[4]

Sexual selection is based on the principal that those members of a species who display features that translate fitness become the most sexually sought after. Thereby, those genes will be most favored in the mating game. If a female cardinal has evolved the notion that a really red male is the most desirable, she will go for the reddest cock she can find. But the most fascinating thing about this type of sexual selection is that when sexual traits are the ones being selected by members of a species, the force of evolution is no longer a random act shaped by mere survival. Intelligent choices are being made and exerted that shape the way a species evolves. This is selective breeding, similar to the way in which dog breeders have created everything from the Great Dane to the Labradoodle from wolf stock. Through sexual selection animal species are altered by animal minds and the choices they make, and this includes the minds of *our* ancient ancestors, who by their sexual preferences created us. We are the end product of what they deemed desirable, just like a rhino is the end product of what its ancestors found attractive—a horn made of hair. And most of this choosing was done by females over every species, and for this reason, that females had so much power, scientists tended to disregard the great power of sexual selection, paying little attention to Darwin's solution until recently.

THE SEXIEST ANIMALS

Zoologist Desmond Morris calls humans the "sexiest animals alive." Nature has given us the hard-wiring we need for sex to be foremost in our brains, and once the hormones kick in at adolescence our minds are abducted with dreams of dating and mating until the eventual point of reproduction occurs, at which time we then have to deal with the huge task of raising our progeny. Unlike other mammals, human females are receptive to sexual intercourse all year round, even when they are not fertile. In most species, a female comes into "heat" only at specific times of the year, during which time she signals through scent or visual stimuli—like the swollen sex glands of female chimps—that she is ovulating and ready to mate. But in humans ovulation is masked. We make a perpetual activity of sex—regardless of the calendar. As we age, sexuality continues for humans even into the eighties (marriage greatly facilitates this, with a greater decline for women than men). For men, sexual interest fades little (even if they are aging and experiencing erectile dysfunction—hence the booming profits of Viagra). And even though some women, as young as in their thirties and forties, report that they are no longer interested in sex once they are done desiring more children, at the same time most of these women will spend fortunes on products to keep them looking young, which from an evolutionary perspective equals giving off the right symbols of our species that imply fertility and sexual attractiveness. Women *do not* want to give up on love, and these beauty products are used as ways of tricking the male brain. Louann Brizendine, in *The Female Brain*, states that

> worldwide, men prefer physically attractive wives, between ages twenty and forty, who are on average of two and a half years younger than they are. They also want potential long-term mates to have clear skin, bright eyes, full lips, shiny hair, and curvy, hourglass figures. The fact that these mate preferences hold true in every culture indicates that they're part of men's hardwired inheritance from their ancient forefathers. . . .
>
> Why would these particular criteria top men's lists? From a practical perspective, all of these traits, superficial as they may seem, are strong visual markers of fertility. Whether or not men know it consciously, their brains know that female fertility offers them the biggest reproductive payoff for their investment . . . over millions of years, male brain wiring

evolved to scan women for quick visual clues to their fertility. Age, of course, is one important factor; health is another. A high activity level, youthful gait, symmetrical physical features, smooth skin, lustrous hair, and lips plumped by estrogen are easily observable signs of age, fertility, and health. So it's no wonder women are reaching for the plumping effects of collagen injections and the wrinkle smoothing of Botox.[5]

Even if it's not a conscious decision for sex per se, the underlying motivation for keeping as far as possible from showing signs of aging is to attract.

The whole business of being sexy for our species starts at puberty, or a few years before, when many girls begin to use cosmetics to enhance their natural physical attractors: such as lipstick (which has been used since ancient times). Desmond Morris theorizes that plump red lips (further exaggerated through additional artificial highlighting of them through cosmetics) physically mimics the labia, which during sexual activity becomes flushed with blood. "This is not, of course, a conscious imitation of the genital signals; it is merely 'sexy' or 'attractive.'"[6] The swollen breasts of female humans are another sexual attractor that begins to develop at puberty, something other primates lack. Chimps and gorillas have pronounced breasts only during lactation (apparently there is no relation between milk production and breast size) and most of the time are flat-chested. Human females display hemispherically rounded breasts constantly, due to genetically developed fat deposits. The female buttocks also undergo expansion during puberty (this in line with the more ancient display of the rump region, central for mating for all mammals except humans and bonobo chimps who, like humans, can also mate face to face). Once again, this is due to fat reserves that build up the buttocks at puberty. In Victorian times, the female bustle was a cultural exaggeration of the buttocks, while in other cultures, such as the Bushmen of Southern Africa, sexual selection has caused a condition known as steatopygia, in which the buttocks of the women are extremely pronounced and protruding, due to genetic selection, as if these women were wearing a bustle. For females around the world, body hair is also much less pronounced than that of men.

Men have evolved their own sexual attractors, such as facial hair, a strong jaw-line, greater height and musculature, a deep voice, and an Adam's apple, caused by testosterone released in the womb shortly after birth and then later at puberty. In addition, because of our upright stance, the penis of male humans is displayed, which in other primates is usually not. Like us, in most other primates the penis is not endowed with any particular markings, though there are a few primates who do display it proudly and in bright color, such as the Mandrill Baboon. However, the codpiece, (or braguette in French) originating in the fifteenth century and lasting for two hundred years in fashion, was a cultural ornament of clothing employed in men's pantaloons, originally as a flap that allowed men to urinate without removing their trousers, that quickly escalated into a fashion rage that included wildly protruding exaggerations of male genitalia of a variety of shapes that were even worn by royalty of various European countries. The greatest difference in the human male penis to other species, though, comes from the fact it does not contain a penis bone, as is found in most all mammals (which allows for an instant erection). Consequently, copulation for humans has taken a quite different turn, with sexual arousal becoming much less mechanical in our species and of much greater duration. At the same time, the penis is much wider and longer than in either chimps or gorillas, and able to stimulate female orgasms (a sexually selected trait, as human females over time preferred such peni). Human females are also endowed with a clitoris and the ability to have orgasms, something that our female primate cousins do not exhibit.

ORNAMENTAL MIND

Geoffrey Miller came up with a theory of the Ornamental Mind, which he developed after rethinking Darwin's work regarding sexual selection. Miller believes that being endowed with brains that give us the ability to create infinitely flexible languages with copious vocabularies and artistic achievements of an endless variety—music, literature, ritual, drama, comedy, monumental architecture, and technology—as well as to partake in the daily range of emotions and thoughts—humor, empathy, sympathy, kindness, charity, religious thought—means that something was at work in our ancient ancestors that went far beyond such abilities in other primate species. "To Darwin, high cost, apparent uselessness, and manifest beauty usually indicated that a behavior had a hidden courtship function."[7] The Ornamental Mind Theory states that not only are the arts (including language and music) products of sexual selection, but so is the human brain itself. Our ancient ancestors, like all animals, were making decisions regarding mates. Females desired males who were tall, fast, strong, and dominant; males desired females who were youthful and fertile. But other traits were selected because they seemed sexy and desirable—the ability to make music, eventually speech itself, the ability to make nice things out of wood or rock, to crack a joke, to keep life from being a bore. Humans desired keen intelligence in other humans, as well as beauty and grace. Miller believes that sexual selection is the primary force that drove human intelligence, as choices were continually being made that led to smarter offspring: in the same way that peahens made choices leading to larger tails in peacocks. But in our species, men as well as women found big brains attractive, and relationships between males and females would alter drastically, giving both genders an equal footing when it came to intelligence.

Howard Hughes medical researchers have recently discovered hundreds to thousands of genetic changes "were acquired during the mere twenty to twenty-five million years of time in the evolutionary lineage leading to humans," and "that selection has worked 'extra-hard' during human evolution to create the powerful" brains we have. Great leaps were made with "the appearance of the genus Homo about 2 million years ago, a major expansion of the brain beginning about a half million years ago, and the appearance of anatomically modern humans about 150,000 years ago."[8]

A number of other physical forces had to alter as brain size increased, including the problem of delivery for the upright hominid female. Pregnancy is and always has been dangerous to women, for any number of problems can put the mother's life at risk. As our ancestors went from walking like chimps and gorillas (knuckle-walkers) to standing up, enormous pressures were put upon the female body that made giving birth much more difficult than it had ever been before. As the brains of infants got larger, things got even worse. The pelvis could physically not become wider if women were to be able to walk on two legs. So the solution was for the infant to be born prematurely in order to make it through the woman's pelvis. But growing that massive brain outside the womb also meant that the human child would be helpless for many years.

In most mammals it is the female, solely, who raises the young. But with children now dependent for years upon parents for sustenance, like many birds, our species began pair-bonding. Females needed help to make sure those children would survive. Those women with mates who stayed around to help raise the kids had a tremendous advantage, since it now took fifteen or more years for a child to become an adult. So women (like female birds) had to be very picky in their mating preferences, and it was advantageous for them to seek qualities in males that not only showed vigor, dominance, and strength, but also kindness and loyalty. Since males were more heavily invested in raising their helpless offspring, to make sure their DNA survived, and were now pair-bonding with females, they also began to seek kind and loving qualities in their mates, with whom they were now closely allied over a number of years. But while sexual selection can drive evolution it cannot create perfection, and every change is forged from a previous trait. Trickster tales reveal the fact that while we are capable of love and fidelity (in many stories Trickster has a wife), the underlying forces of promiscuity did not go away. Both from the male trickster perspective, of unleashed sexual appetite, to the female trickster, who must outwit the continual pawing and manipulation of the male, more than any other theme, trickster stories revolve around sex.

6

THE BRAIN OF LOVE AND WAR

Everything human is pathetic. The secret source of Humor itself is
not joy but sorrow. There is no humor in heaven.

—Mark Twain

David Buss's study of thirty-seven cultures found that "kindness" was
the number one desired trait worldwide by both men and women when
selecting a mate. Sex not dependent upon ovulation, with sexual access
available year-round, added emotional force to pair-bonding, while
kindness made the likelihood that a pair-bond would last at least long
enough to get the child on its feet. For males, the question of paternity
for pair-bonded animals is always a central concern (for males do not
want to invest in someone else's DNA), and emotional jealousy developed in humans as a way of controlling females, who now showed no
signs for when they were fertile. For males, it was important that no
cheating was going on. But from the female's perspective, to lose a
valuable mate to another female would also have had devastating consequences in terms of her ability to raise offspring (just as in pair-bonded
birds)—even if that meant having to share resources with a second lover
or wife. So jealousy arose in females as well as a way of limiting male
philandering. With an actual pair-bonded relationship now taking place

over years instead of days, males and females both became choosier in the new paradigm of hooking up, and those choices had profound consequences for the mating ritual.

The courtship process became longer and more intense, with language, music, and all the arts playing a role in attracting and wooing a member of the opposite sex. Biologically, our bodies changed from hairy to hairless, and our overall physical appearance was revolutionized from that of an ape to a *Homo erectus* (tall, lean, muscular, who resembled us quite closely, even though their brain sizes were still half of ours today). One branch of *Homo erectus* eventually evolved into us. Nowadays, it is known that evolution works not only through slow progression, but also in starts and fits, with organisms existing for long periods of time in a state of equilibrium, while at other times evolution erupts with great genetic mutation and change within isolated populations (keep in mind that we're still talking about tens of thousand of years). This scenario is exactly what occurred during the Pleistocene, which lasted from 1.6 million years ago to 10,000 years ago, when we went from being ape-like hominids to human beings (Homo sapiens emerging some 200,000 to 150,000 years ago in Africa).

Numerous changes occurred in our species between men and women as our ancestors developed the repertoire of behaviors we think of as human, but there was never a Golden Age in which men and women were without strife. The cobbled-together evolution of our trickster brains prevented that. As mentioned previously, men and women have had some unusual evolutionary trajectories since the sexes in our species took on specialized kinds of work. For millennia, men have spent much of their time hunting for meat, while women have spent much of their time gathering foodstuff and raising children. Sexual selection and natural selection created different qualities for males and females that portrayed "fitness." And even though some qualities for altruistic behavior within the pair-bond and group were especially being selected for, this did not mean that qualities of male aggression and dominance were bred completely out of our species. Males who displayed greater athleticism in hunting and warfare and who were dominant within the hierarchy of the tribe were still seen as being overall the most attractive mates. This is borne out in ethnological studies of contemporary tribal people, with tribal leaders usually having not only more resources but the most wives. Attitudes regarding mate choice can also be seen through psychological studies of contemporary people around the world in every culture, regardless of political or educational factors:

> Women in the overwhelming majority of cultures value ambition and industry more than men do, typically rating it as between important and indispensable. . . . This cross-cultural and cross-time evidence supports the key evolutionary expectation that women have evolved a preference for men who show signs of the ability to acquire resources and a disdain for men who lack ambition. This preference helped ancestral women to solve the critical adaptive problem of obtaining reliable resources. . . . a man's ambition and industriousness provided a guarantee of the continuation of those resources.[1]

Though pair-bonding and the possibility for altruistic behavior came into our species through sexual selection, it was never a perfect system. Not only did suspicion of outsiders and perpetual warfare become a hallmark of our species, the "war between men and women," as cartoonist James Thurber put it back in the 1930s, never subsided. Pair-bonding, and everything that surrounds it, such as notions of monogamy, marriage, paternity, property, and so on, developed over the much more ancient wiring for promiscuity.

MONOGAMY?

To answer the question of monogamy, anthropologists have looked to our closest cousins for answers. One clue can be gleaned through sperm. It turns out there are three different kinds of sperm, which have evolved for a reason. Some sperm lock tails and form a chastity belt around the egg, while other sperm turn into what look like little Pac-Men—hunting out alien sperm and murdering them. Then there are the actual mating sperm, who must also get through the chastity-belt sperm, but *they can* because the chastity-belt sperm will recognize these fellow sperm as swimming from their own home team and will let one of them pass. But if another man's sperm tries to make his way in, forget it. There's no way the foreign sperm is going to squirm past the bouncers. The other guy's sperm contains alien DNA that the chastity-belt sperm can recognize at once. All of this evidence, of course, implies that monogamy was not part of our ancient ancestors, for this sperm defense system would never have developed if monogamy had been part of our ancient past.[2]

Another clue regarding past sexual practices in our ancient ancestors lies in the size of a male's scrotum. In chimpanzees, where sex is mostly a free-for-all (with the most dominant getting the preferential advantage), males have massive testicles and incredible ejaculatory power, for males are in direct competition with other males to get their sperm into an egg. Since all the males have some possibility of access to ovulating females, having larger testicles and more sperm increases their chances for success (dominant chimps still get preferential treatment sexually). Gorillas, who are much larger than chimps, have teeny testicles, for they live in harems in which the males do not have to worry about other males mating with their female consorts. The testicles of humans are right in between in size, with the implications being that our ancient mating system was mixed—just as it is today.

Monogamy is extremely rare in primates and exists in none of our closest relatives. The only physical evidence from the past regarding sexual strategies comes from looking at the fossil record for sexual dimorphism (the size difference between males and females). In species, such as the gorilla, where the male is greatly larger than the female, the mating pattern is that of a harem. Among chimpanzees, in which there is male dominance, but no harem, there is greater sexual dimorphism than in humans, but not nearly as much as in gorillas, and in the bonobo (a more gracile sub-species of chimp) there is even less. Generally, the more monogamous the species the more the males and females will be the same size. Human males are slightly larger than females, indicating the kind of mating behavior attested to from other research—a mix of pair-bonding and promiscuity, polygyny, and monogamy.

Bonobos are a close relative who have sex continually (the trickster's ideal). They are the only other primates, besides us, who can have face-to-face sex, and they indulge in the pleasures of sex at every opportunity in unlimited ways. Also, in bonobo society, females, in particular, form alliances with one another, which keeps dominant males in check. At any hint of stress within a troop, sex is initiated, which can be between males and males, males and females, females and females, young and old. In comparison to common chimps, from the human standpoint, there is a lot in bonobo society that seems preferable—greatly lessened male brutality, dominance, and violence. When news of bonobo behavior first entered the mainstream, a number of feminists were heartened that an ape cousin had been discovered who displayed a more egalitarian societal model in which females were not the second-rate citizens they were in common chimp society. But further investigation has shown that there is really no reason to think that the bonobo model existed as a template for our direct line of ape ancestors. Neither human pair-bonding nor harem-like configuration have anything to do with the bonobo world, and the environment of thick jungle (and the consequent evolutionary pressures from that particular environment) was quite opposite of our savannah living relations who long before becoming homo sapiens most likely lived in male-dominated polygynous relationships.

Even now, an examination of societies around the globe has led most researchers to conclude that polygyny (multiple sexual partners for men) tends to slightly edge out monogamy. As G. A. Schuiling states in "The Benefit and the Doubt: Why Monogamy?" "For humans, the optimal evolutionary strategy is monogamy when necessary, polygamy when possible."[3] Pair-bonding, when it began in our ancestors, was most likely serial monogamy, with cheating. For it is polygyny that fuels sexual selection to a much greater extent than monogamy can. And if all the traits we think of as defining our "humanity" were highly influenced by sexual selection, as Miller contends, polygyny helps explain how such changes could sweep so quickly through our ancestors when Homo sapiens arose. Recent scientific study of molecular genetic data, "based on up to 166 Y-chromosome SNPs, in 46 samples from all continents," also suggests that the movement from polygyny to monogamy was very recent:

> Until recently only a few men may have contributed a large fraction of the Y-chromosome pool at every generation. The number of breeding males may have increased, and the variance of their reproductive success may have decreased, through a recent shift from polygyny to monogamy, which is supported by ethnological data and possibly accompanied the shift from mobile to sedentary communities.[4]

So, pair-bonding developed on top of the much older instinct for promiscuity, but just like in bird species today is a strategy filled with strife.

If it had been perfect, the cultural institution of marriage would have had no need to have arisen to act as a societal brake on promiscuous sexual behavior.

In contemporary hunting and gathering tribal societies, a man having more than one wife is relatively uncommon, outside of headmen or chiefs, for there is little chance in these reciprocal societies for any wealth to be developed (status is determined through hunting ability or personal charisma), but as soon as some wealth or power can be accumulated, the situation changes dramatically. It should be mentioned, however, that even in polygamous societies, marriage exists, with legal status usually belonging to the first wife only. Marriage is universal for our species, and polygyny (a man with more than one sexual partner—who may also have an official wife) is more common than polygamy (a man with numerous wives). Polyandry, in which a woman has multiple husbands, is so rare as to be statistically insignificant. What these arrangements mean in terms of the psychological effects they might have for the women and men involved is very difficult to ascertain and to a certain extent dependent upon cultural mores and interpretation.

WOMEN AND WAR

The anthropological evidence from tribal societies appears to be that when it comes to gender behavior, exploitation of women is not a general case. In these societies, with their division of labor, where men do the hunting and the women the gathering and child-rearing, there is difference but relative equality. As Desmond Morris says, "It's almost certain that throughout our long evolutionary past, that the human animal has thrived on this natural balance of power between the sexes, rather than the domination of one sex by the other."[5] These primal societies are called "egalitarian," because there is food sharing between all members, with no *formal* hierarchical structure. Therefore, no individual has any political authority over another, though of course dominant personalities arise within these cultures who can become powerful leaders. Yet, men still retain more political power than women. Within the domains of separate male and female social systems there are also status rankings as well, just as occur in chimpanzee and bonobo societies.

In tribal life, men vie for the "most fit" females they can attract, and women vie for the "most fit" males, with sometimes fierce competition for mates between both sexes. Men bond with one another through their hunting activities and totem societies, and women bond through child-raising and gathering. Women spend much more time communicating with other women through spoken language during the course of their daily jobs. And within the tribe, there are often great displays of kindness between all members. Sexual love plays a large part with courting couples, and familial love plays a large part with family and other tribal members. This is reflected in the name most tribal people have for themselves, which would translate as "the humans beings." It sounds very inclusive and loving, but upon closer examination we see that the implications are that if one is not part of the tribe, one is not quite human. Within the tribe, women tend to be best at conflict resolution, expressing fewer violent tendencies. While men tend to be about twenty times more aggressive than women, most of this tends to be directed to non-tribal members, as there are strict taboos against full-fledged inner-tribal violence. This doesn't mean that dominance struggles don't occur in both sexes, for they can erupt between men and between women. For this reason, many cultures have developed avoidance taboos to limit this (some people who live in intimate conditions, such as a man and his mother-in-law in the same tepee, are not allowed to speak to one another).

Interestingly enough, warfare between tribes, throughout the world, has most often been motivated by the desire of men from one tribe to steal the women of another. As Buss says,

> Among the Yanomamo, there are two key motives that spur men to declare war on another tribe—a desire to capture the wives of other men or a desire to recapture wives that were lost in previous raids. When the American anthropologist Napoleon Chagnon explained to his Yanomamo informants that his country declared war for ideals such as freedom and democracy, they were astonished. It seemed silly to them to risk one's life for anything other than capturing women.[6]

This brings up the long-standing assumption in anthropology that primal/tribal societies led basically peaceful lives, and that warfare, when it existed, was essentially a sport in which few were killed. Anthropologists of the past saw warfare as a kind of game that was only the surface result of deeper needs for nutritional resources. This interpretation was highly influenced by the definition of human nature developed by Jean-Jacques Rousseau (1712–1778), who believed that humans were basically noble, and in the natural state of primitive man could be found the most exemplary examples of humankind, people untouched by the avarice of civilization, with its greed and corruption. (Jean Thomas Hobbes, 1588–1679, earlier, and on the opposite end of the spectrum, believed that human nature was brutish and cruel).

However, Lawrence H. Keeley shows, convincingly, in his book *War Before Civilization*, that warfare has been a constant of nearly every primal society around the world, and that rather than being sport, primitive warfare was highly aggressive, brutal, and deadly, occurring even more frequently in tribal cultures than some later state-level societies with their full-time armies and dedicated machinery for war. At the same time, this does not mean that man is essentially as Hobbes described, for people everywhere are highly influenced by culture, as the non-warlike Swedes of today are descended from the notorious Vikings who raped and pillaged Europe for centuries. Likewise, the Mongols of Genghis Khan have turned into Buddhists. What the evidence does show, though, is that there is always a danger for war to exist in human societies, primarily because of the psychological condition of young men, who are highly susceptible to group-think and easily coerced into regimented behavior. As Morris states, it is the "acceptance of group orders that can lead to the horrors of warfare. War is more the result of male group cooperation than it is male aggression. The soldier kills more to conform and support his buddies than for his personal hatred of the enemy."[7] Human beings are highly influenced by social custom in general, especially young men, and this paired with the fact that the brain does not mature fully until the age of twenty-five, means that young men, fueled by testosterone, can easily be both seduced into the glory of war and led into submission by strong commanders. As anyone who has read about war knows, it is young men who have marched head on into the most foolhardy and hopeless situations (in today's armies, of course, we also see women marching into the battlefields).

But for women, sexual exploitation is still the monstrous currency of war—even today—from Sarajevo to the Congo to Darfur, both a tactic and a motivation for war. Lawrence H. Keeley states that in tribal societies

> the capture of women was one of the spoils of victory—and occasionally one
> of the primary aims of warfare—for many tribal warriors. In many societies, if the men lost a fight, the women were subject to capture and forced
> incorporation into the captor's society. Most Indian tribes in western North
> America at least occasionally conducted raids to capture women. The social
> position of captive women varied widely among cultures, from abject slaves
> to concubines to secondary wives to full spouses. In a few cases, female
> captives could be ransomed or, of course, escape. In situations where ransom or escape were not possible, the treatment of captive young women
> amounted to rape, whether actual violence was used against them to enforce cohabitation with their captors or was only implicit in their situation.[8]

Nicholas Wade raises the point that historians are often loath to attribute evolutionary pressures as a cause for wars and conquest, but in this
they may just be not looking at the evidence:

> Sexual Selection . . . the effort by one male to propagate his genes at the
> expense of others, has been a powerful force throughout primate history,
> from chimpanzee societies to those of the Yanomamo [South American
> Indians who admit that warfare is collecting females. It has operated
> with little change in more complex societies, especially during times
> when access to women was one of the accepted rewards of power. Even
> in many contemporary societies, where at least a pretense of monogamy
> is expected of rulers, the old instincts have not disappeared [here Wade
> mentions Chairman Mao]. . . .
>   Presidents John F. Kennedy and Bill Clinton conducted affairs while
> serving in the White House. "I don't know of a single head of state who
> hasn't yielded to some kind of carnal temptation, small or large. That in
> itself is a reason to govern," said Francois Mitterrand, the French president. . . . Perhaps the brute desire to procreate might drive the affairs of
> state is a concept that historians find too gross to contemplate.[9]

Within their own group, most hunting-gathering society tribal women
were most likely essentially equal with men. But as terrorism was always a
threat, through raiding, rape, and kidnapping, the traditional portrayal of
tribal life as idyllic is obviously just another case of Edenic mythologizing.

CIVILIZATION AND ENSLAVEMENT OF WOMEN

Contrary to what most believe, many of our species—*but especially women*—paid a very high price for living within the great cultural changes of "civilization," even when accounting for tribal warfare over women. Humans were bred through natural and sexual selection to exist within small tribal units, but now our biology ran straight into conflict with the new technologies of agriculture and state-level society. With the rise of the first permanent settlements about 10,000 years ago came the development of writing as specialized knowledge available only to the elite; formal hierarchy and caste systems with highly structured political power; formal religious organizations and a priestly caste in control of ritual, social law, and access to the gods; specialization of workers (farmers, artisans, soldiers, police); the accumulation of stuff: everything from architecture to furniture and clothing; and standing armies to protect all that stuff and to go to war to steal it from others. Human beings were now subjected to authority and forced to work in ways they could never have imagined in tribal life. For in hunting and gathering societies there is no "boss," and the efforts to maintain life often take a minimal amount of time each day (contrary to the usual assumption that civilization gave us leisure). "Work," as we think of it nowadays, was not even a concept with tribal people, who could get by with about twenty hours of effort per week to secure their living. With the accumulation of stuff and power, the roles of men and women changed. Men with power could now enslave women as wives and concubines, and women in certain cultures could be bought and sold as chattel. Formal misogyny against women was part of the shift from tribal culture that took various forms—from brutal to subtle—leaving many women in civilized cultures as second-class citizens or worse.

In tribal societies that have agriculture or herding, where wealth can be accumulated, about three-fourths are polygamous, for having more than one wife requires an excess of resources (those men without wealth often must remain celibate). Even in modern civilizations, where monogamy is enforced as the only legal mating arrangement allowed by the government, many men are still involved in serial monogamy—where an individual has numerous partners, consecutively, over the course of a lifetime, and it is often wealth that allows those practices for men to occur. But in outright polygamous cultures, the number of sexual partners for males with power could be staggering. King Solomon, in the Old Testament is said in the Bible to have had 700 wives and 300 concubines, which Mark Twain, in great trickster fashion, brings up in *The Adventures of Huckleberry Finn*, when Huck and Jim share this exchange:

> [Huck] "The place where he keeps his wives. Don't you know about the harem? Solomon had one; he had about a million wives."
> [Jim] "Why, yes, dat's so; I—I'd done forgot it. A harem's a bo'd'n-house, I reck'n. Mos' likely dey has rackety times in de nussery. En I reck'n de wives quarrels considable; en dat 'crease de racket. Yit dey say Sollermun de wises' man dat ever live'. I doan' take no stock in dat. Bekase why would a wise man want to live in de mids' er sich a blim-blammin' all de time?"[10]

The Bible's claim may seem nothing more than hyperbole, but those numbers are in line with what is known about many other rulers. Genghis Khan, for example, had 500 wives and an endless number of concubines, and what DNA studies have shown recently are astounding: "8 percent of males throughout the former lands of the Mongol empire carry the Y chromosome of Genghis Khan. This amounts to a total of 16 million men, or about 0.5 percent of the world's total."[11] Further examples of royal sexual proclivity are just as mind-boggling:

> The Babylonian king Hammurabi had thousands of slave wives at his command. The Egyptian pharaoh Akhenaton procured 317 concubines and "droves" of consorts. The Aztec ruler Montezuma enjoyed 4,000 concubines. The Indian emperor Udayama preserved sixteen thousand consorts in apartments ringed by fire and guarded by eunuchs. The Chinese emperor Fei-ti had ten thousand women in his harem.[12]

History is loaded with emperors, kings, and rulers of every stripe who have indulged in sexual excess, and this tradition continues in parts of the world where royal harems are still allowed.

But men in state-level societies also lived miserable and futile lives, as serfs, soldiers, and slaves. Class distinctions made all the difference in the kind of life one could expect to have, and over time differing societies developed different norms for how men and women should be treated, which usually depended upon one's station in society. While in most cases women of any strata within civilized society were seen as inferior to men (here, leaving out the great women monarchs—the true exceptions), the differences in how women lived and were treated at the top compared to the bottom of society could be the difference between heaven and hell.

WHY LOVE?

This brings us to the heart. Love. Why did love evolve within our species? Attachment and bonding can be seen in many animals, across numerous species. But in our species love has developed to an extreme degree. The answer to "why love" is directly tied to paternity. When females give birth there is no question of who the mother is, but there is always a question of who donated the sperm. In the animal world, this drive to be sure that the male's progeny actually carry his DNA creates behavior such as male lions killing the cubs of any female when he moves into a pride, or of a bull elk herding the cows during rutting season to make sure they don't stray. Any kind of harem situation in which the male guards against other male suitors is because of paternity, be they gorillas, baboons, or any of thousands of other species. In monogamous bonds, be it birds or gibbons, paternity is the primary question as well. As mentioned before, our species developed strategies against cheating, and love is one of those strategies.

Before getting to the point of making love (of course) we have to eat, and nearly all courtship rituals revolve around this bonding device: a male offering a present of food, as in the first date dinner, or even going out for a cup of coffee—interestingly enough, for many bird species a gift of food is the first courting ritual as well. An expression of art (in the form of going to a movie or a concert, bringing a flower) is another (the Bowerbird exhibits the closest animal behavior to art creation in the world, as it builds monumental architectural nests for courtship). In humans, courtship also equals extreme verbal displays. Evidence shows that a couple will utter 1,000,000 words each before conceiving (once again, some birds learn, or make up, a thousand or more songs with which to court). Miller, in answering critics' charges against language as stemming from courtship ritual, states, "Human verbal courtship is the least superficial form of courtship that evolution has ever produced. A million words give a panoramic view of someone's personality, past, plans, hopes, fears and ideals."[13]

We humans undergo an elaborate courtship ritual more extravagant than even whooping cranes. And though there are cultural variations, love is a universal phenomenon of human experience. Desmond Morris pointed out years ago that love *is a biological adaptation*, not just an element of culture. Love is also a universal phenomenon, not just a luxuriously decadent pastime of Western culture, as was once claimed. For while we know that love is the subject of most popular songs in the West, and we are used to hearing love songs in every musical genre— folk, jazz, blues, rock—many have not seen love as the universal attribute of human behavior it is. Love, sex, and marriage are played out so differently in various cultures, the tendency has been to deny the biology of love.

Part of this goes back to racist notions that dark-skinned people were incapable of romantic love: another convenient excuse to justify slavery and exploitation. It was often impossible for Westerners to attribute such fully "human" characteristics to Others, even well into the twentieth century. In addition, the arranged marriages of many cultures seemed the antithesis of romantic love to those of us in the West, further supporting the idea that "those people" could not possibly know what it means to *fall in love*. Books like *Love in the Western World, The Hoax of Romance*, and James Parks' "Romantic Love Is a Hoax! Emotional Programming to 'Fall in Love'" proposed that romantic love was cultural and (as Parks says) did not exist until as recently as 800 years ago. This idea actually became prevalent in parts of academia, where love was sometimes seen as just a decadent bourgeois affliction of a bored middle class, heightened by Hollywood. But those assessments were wrong.

What is love? It's still a good question. Our usual concept of "falling in love" includes a deep desire for attachment that hits like lightning, enveloping the whole self, desiring constant togetherness, as a powerful feeling invades every aspect of the body and mind. Research in neuroscience has now completely shifted the view on love. Anthropologist Helen Fisher (who has devoted years to the study, cross-culturally) says that we have "evolved a specific brain network" which has created an innate "circuitry for love."[14] Likewise, Louann Brizendine, in *The Female Brain*, says that what we have is "the brain architecture of love, engineered by the reproductive winners in evolution. Even the shapes, faces, smells, and ages of the mates we choose are influenced by patterns set millennia ago."[15] There are stages of love that most people of all cultures pass through, based upon pre-wiring in the brain, and neuroscience has been able to unlock both the chemical underpinnings of love and well as revealing mental maps of love through MRI scans.

Larry Young, in *Nature*, states that

we are not alone in being able to form intense and enduring social ties. Take the mother–infant bond. Whether or not the emotional connection between a ewe and her lamb, or a female macaque and her offspring, is qualitatively similar to human motherly love, it is highly likely that these relationships share evolutionarily conserved brain mechanisms. In humans, rats and sheep, the hormone oxytocin is released during labor, delivery and nursing. In ewes, an infusion of oxytocin into the brain results in rapid bonding with a foreign lamb.

Long-term bonding between mates is rare in mammals. It may be regulated by the same brain mechanisms as those involved in maternal bonding. For instance, pair bonding in the female monogamous prairie vole is stimulated by oxytocin released in the brain during mating. A female prairie vole rapidly becomes attached to the nearest male if her brain is infused with oxytocin. [It should be noted here that prairie vole males with naturally raised levels of vasopressin are monogamous, but those with little are not]. The hormone interacts with the reward and reinforcement system driven by the neurotransmitter dopamine—the same circuitry that drugs such as nicotine, cocaine and heroine act on in humans to produce euphoria and addiction.[16]

THE POWER OF LOVE: WOMEN'S SONGS OF LOVE FROM AFGHANISTAN

A remarkable collection (*Songs of Love and War*) of contemporary songs from Afghan women who are forced into arranged marriages, whose husbands and sons beat them, and who are made to work in the most incomprehensible conditions where no love exists, shows that even in such a deadening culture where women are never exposed to models of romantic love there is still an incredible longing for it. In this culture, where women see their only way out as suicide, they still write wrenching love songs that almost always describe illicit affairs, defying all the powers that be and putting themselves in jeopardy:

> You were hiding behind the door,
> I was stroking my naked breasts and you caught sight of me.
>
> I will gladly give you my mouth,
> But why stir my pitcher? Here I am now, all wet.
>
> First take me into your arms and hold me close,
> Only then will you be able to join my velvet thighs.

Current science shows that our desire for and reasons for selecting mates involves much more than "rational" choices consciously made by family members or the lovers themselves. These songs attest to the more powerful and ancient set of biological impulses that are set in motion during puberty. A longing for romantic love is a universal human phenomenon. While love is built upon the brain-wiring foundations for attachment we see in other animals, in humans that neural wiring has been altered over thousands of generations to become unique. It is nature's way of flooding the brain with chemicals for both mating and attachment, leading to a kind of intimacy that goes far beyond anything else in the animal world. But it's a game of high stakes, constant assessment and reassessment, a psychological thriller full of paranoia, all-consuming lust, jealousy, and madness. As Shakespeare said, "If thou remember'st not the slightest folly/That ever love did make thee run into/ Thou hast not loved." Shakespeare constantly parodied the insanity of love in his plays, from *Romeo and Juliet* to *Twelfth Night*, showing us in dramatic form the fools we can become. Anthropologist Helen Fisher describes falling in love as having the following characteristics:

1. Concentration—a love object that takes on "special meaning."
2. Focused Attention—at this point, other potential mating partners are locked out, and a laser focus is directed toward one individual.

3. Aggrandizing the Beloved—magnifying the positive aspects of the loved one.
4. Intrusive Thinking—obsession over the loved one.
5. Emotional Fire—intense passion and emotional response.
6. Intense Energy.
7. Mood Swings—from ecstasy to despair.
8. Yearning for Emotional Union.
9. Looking for Clues—hypersensitivity to what the beloved is thinking about the lover.
10. Changing Priorities—new clothing styles, working out, new interests.
11. Emotional Dependence—including separation anxiety.
12. Empathy—for the beloved.
13. Adversity Heightens Passion—in which anything preventing the lovers from uniting adds fuel to the flame—social standing, travel, work, etc.
14. Hope—not giving up, even if things begin to take a bad turn.
15. A Sexual Connection.
16. Sexual Exclusivity.
17. Jealousy.
18. Emotional Union Trumps Sexual Union.
19. Involuntary, Uncontrollable Love—no logical control over the relationship.
20. A Transient State—the rollercoaster cannot go on indefinitely— "a team of neuroscientists recently concluded that romantic love normally lasts between twelve and eighteen months."[17]

The neurochemicals of love are more powerful than cocaine or heroin: nature's "trick" for making sure the genes not only perpetuate themselves, but that the two parents stay around long enough to get the child to where it can stand. (Fisher estimates this as being four years, the average time period for mated pairs before divorce in tribal societies around the world, which is just enough time to get the young one to a semi-independent state—no longer demanding 100 percent of a parent's attention.)

Neuroscientist Louann Brizendine agrees with Shakespeare, that love is akin to madness and "infatuation-love is now a documented brain state":

It shares brain circuits with states of obsession, mania, intoxication, thirst, and hunger. It is not an emotion, but it does intensify or decreases other emotions. The being-in-love circuits are primarily a motivation system, which is different from the brain's sex drive area but overlaps with it. This fevered brain activity runs on hormones and neurochemicals such as dopamine, estrogen, oxytocin, and testosterone.

The brain circuits that are activated when we are in love match those of the drug addict desperately craving the next fix. The amygdala—the brain's fear-alert system—and the anterior cingulated cortex—the brain's worry and critical thinking system—are turned way down when the love circuits are running full blast. Much the same thing happens when people take Ecstasy: the normal wariness humans have toward strangers is switched off and the love circuits are dialed up. So romantic love is a natural Ecstasy high. The classic symptoms of early love are also similar to the initial effects of drugs such as amphetamines, cocaine, and opiates like heroin, morphine, and oxytocin. These narcotics trigger the brain's reward circuit, causing chemical releases and effects similar to those of romance. In fact, there's some truth to the notion that people can become addicted to love. Romantic partners, especially in the first six months, crave the ecstatic feeling of being together and may feel helplessly depen-dent on each other . . . . This is such an intense state that the beloved's best interest, well-being, and survival become as important as or more important than one's own.[18]

As most of us know, sexual love can be very dangerous, and while it is something that every human craves, it is risk-taking behavior that can have huge consequences—not the least of which is caring for the child that may ensue.

The superb film *Fast Runner* is a perfect example of how love and lust can create all that is needed for high drama. Set in the Arctic Circle in ancient times, this mythic Inuit story (filmed entirely with Inuit actors) involves two brothers and jealousy, as one brother "covets" the other's wife. In the end this jealousy leads to murder and evil, as darkness sweeps through the isolated Inuit villages. The most amazing thing about the story is how all of this drama takes place in an environment where there is physically nothing but ice, snow, and raw seal to eat. Yet, even in such a poor physical culture, the same old story plays out—a story that could have been written in ancient Sumeria 5,000 years ago, by Shakespeare 400 years ago, or David Kelly today. We are the most sophisticated, urbane, educated people who ever lived on earth, yet scratch below the surface and we have the same emotional nervous systems of our ancestors coursing through us, which Trickster is always happy to bring to our attention. For trickster stories quite often touch on the obsessive nature of love and the overwhelming desire for sex. When, for instance, in the Winnebago trickster story, Trickster is supposed to refrain from sexual intercourse before going to war, of course he does the opposite, with the story subtly revealing the connection of war to sexual conquest. In a Nez Perce story Coyote loves his wife so much he cannot refrain from touching her, even though this act banishes her to the land of the dead forever.

7

THE BRAIN OF SONG

It occurred to me by intuition, and music was the driving force behind that intuition. My discovery was the result of musical perception. (When asked about his theory of relativity)

—Albert Einstein

Once language erupted in our species our ancestors' emotional responses to the unexplained mysteries led them to invent the spiritual
universe. Whenever mythic creation first developed in the human mind,
50,000 to 150,000 years ago, it had to have been one of the most momen-
tous times for our species, for here we crossed a divide between life lived
day to day without conscious purpose (though, obviously, a conscious
sense of purpose is not necessary for survival) to a life that is consciously
connected to both a personal historical narrative—language telling the
story of ourselves—to the narrative of the larger social group within an
expanded mythic context. *Aware of being aware* entered our minds,
with the consequent implications of past, present, and future. More and
more questions of "why," must have been formed in our ancestors' heads,
which various people in the community, no doubt, tried to address.

Somewhere in that stir of invention early humans came to see language as a magical force—especially language tied to music: song. Even

in preliterate societies today, language is seen as power, and poetry is always song. Songs are used to do everything from coax the sun up in the morning to sing a child to sleep at night. Song is the primary literary creation of tribal cultures, and it is in song that language is most thoroughly bonded to emotion. It seems likely that the ancients, like tribal people today, evoked song to move the world in the ways that they desired. Song—borne of language and music together—became the first mythic tool.

MUSIC AND LANGUAGE—COMMON ROOTS

Since music and language are the two communicative systems of sequential information in our species, many have theorized on their common root. Many animal species use vocal calls and "songs" to communicate emotions, to signal territorial boundaries, and to alert others to mating readiness. Many of these calls (including those for chimps) are innate, though there is a small degree of individual variation in chimpanzee panting that can be consciously altered by the individual. Yet, some bird species must learn and even *invent* hundreds of songs.[1] Humpbacked whales create songs that are five to twenty minutes long "marked by repeating phrases, rhythm and even rhyme—[which are] sung over and over again for hours."[2] Another form of animal song is chorusing and duetting. Some birds sing in tremendously large choruses, while other birds can duet, "fitting their sounds together so precisely that it is hard to believe that more than one individual is involved."[3] Duetting appears mostly in pair-bonded monogamous birds who hold a specific year-round territory; the reasons why are speculative (this is not the same as synchronous singing). One theory is that the duet enforces the pair-bond, another that these are just territorial calls that a couple is using to defend their territory. In primates, gibbons and siamangs (the only monogamous apes) also sing duets, and they are the only real "singers" in the ape family.

T. Geissmann, who has extensively studied primate vocalizations, says that singing developed a number of times in primate evolution, and that the structure of the singing suggests that singing "evolved each time from loud calls used in a territorial or alarm context" highly emotional in nature.[4] If we look at the nature of song in animal species we can see that it usually functions from emotional stimuli tied to mating, territorial defense, communication with the group, and to intimidate enemies. In other words, singing has very specific purposes and is not done just for the sake of creating interesting effects. (No art for art's sake in the natural world). It is reasonable to think that the same would have applied to our early ancestors: songs would have had specific reasons for existing, and specific meanings would have been conveyed. (I am defining song in the early hominid period as panting, hooting, and rhythmic vocalization). This clearly puts music/song into the adaptive mode—it was serving a purpose and became a selected behavior—helping the survival of individuals.

While music by itself does not have a referential element, as words do, it can still convey referential meaning—especially emotional meaning—everything from "I am free to mate," to "don't step on my turf," "I feel sad, or happy." Within pre-language early hominid groups it seems reasonable to think that vocalizations and rhythms could have eventually gathered greater specificity, possibly standing for more complex thought patterns, such as "there's water over there," or "those guys from the other troop are coming after us—RUN!" This goes back to the concept of schemas, the pre-language thought stories that are at the root of language. Just by looking at the communicative acts of other species, it is clear that rhythm/vocalizations with a musical component came about long before language.

There are many places in which the two systems cross over: both music and language require patterning of sounds that arise from emotional responses. Recall that every thought and utterance is meshed with the oldest emotive parts of the brain: language can never be purely logical and always has an emotional component. In addition, both language and music involve the use of timing, pitch, and tone. The differences are, of course, that music makes us feel, and it is universally understandable (though cultural preferences apply); while language is symbolic, standing for things in the environment as well as abstract ideas. Plus, each language is only comprehensible within its own language community (here, I am eliminating body language and gesture, much of which is universal throughout humans). So, if music and language do come from the same source, at what point, and why, might they have diverged?

TWO CAMPS

There are basically two camps in this debate—emotive and referential. By examining vocal origins through the behavior of living animals, we have just seen how even contemporary animal vocalizations can serve dual purposes—being both emotional and referential—expressing both feeling and concept, and even in our own communication we can see echoes of the pre-vocalization-music/pre-vocalization-language split. When we bark out a warning to someone in danger of being hit by a truck—"Hey!"—it's not so much a word as an exclamation for another to look out (we could also say, "Look Out!" or we could just scream!). When we make the "tsk-tsk" noise to show disapproval, or clear our throats to express our displeasure at another's remark, or expel a burst of air for exasperation—these all show that same pre-language use of sound to convey emotion and meaning. (In the Lakota language, there weren't any swear words, so disgruntlement was expressed by making the bear noise!). When we scream from fear or frustration, or say "ow!" or "ahh!" when stubbing our toe, we are doing something similar, just as we are when laughing, giggling, sobbing, howling, or growling. In addition, we do use musical elements to convey specific meanings: the doorbell rings to signal someone is here; the train whistle alerts us get off the tracks; the tornado alarm warns us to get into a basement; the noon whistle—the school bells ringing—the church bells chiming—all are created to affect our actions; the ice-cream truck's dinging let's us know to run out to the street with a dollar bill.

WHY DID MUSIC AND LANGUAGE SPLIT?

A number of theorists have attempted to go back and look at where and how music and language might have gone their separate ways. One of the most interesting recent discoveries showing the evolutionary link between music and language comes from Dale Purves (a neuroscientist at Duke University) and his colleagues. It has long been known that humans, across cultures, have found the same twelve tones appealing, but as Schwartz, Howe, and Purves state, "The similarity of musical scales and consonance judgments across human populations has no generally accepted explanation."[5] Yet, in August of 2007 Dale Purves discovered that "the tones of the chromatic scale are dominated by the harmonic ratios found in the sound of the human voice." When "tonal intervals, or harmonics, of a single vowel sound were broken down, the frequency ratios of our familiar music scales are usually found."[6] Purves says that this finding calls aesthetics itself into question, stating that "the implicit conclusion in this work is that aesthetics is reduced to biological information, and that is not what musicians and philosophers want to hear."[7] But this is just another corroboration of the evolutionary antecedents of who we are—from music, to language, to art. Here, in this instance, we have the first empirical data linking the physicality of music and language.

Anthropologist Steve Brown developed the Musilanguage concept to explain the origins of music and language, for he says they have the same properties embedded in each other. He carefully goes through the physical steps of how he thinks the two systems, once the same, divided and evolved along parallel lines: lexical units/metrics, propositional syntax/pitch-blending syntax. Brown makes the case that what is often neglected is the fact that there is "musical-language," and "speechmelody," which we now see confirmed in Purves's work. Brown says that

> the phrase is the basic unit of structure and function. It is what makes speaking and singing different from grunting and screaming. In both, a limited repertoire of discrete units is chosen out of an infinite number of possible acoustic elements, such that phrases are generated through combinatorial arrangements of these unitary elements.[8]

Both music and language do contain discreet units that can be combined in numerous ways to produce a variety of "lines." Without punctuation between syllables or notes there would be nothing but nonsense in both music and language. In addition, tonal languages use different pitches to express various meanings for the same sounds, while all languages use tonal variations for emphasis or to shift meaning. "I love you," said flat, without any variation in pitch is not the same thing as "*I* love you," or "I LOVE you," or "I love YOU." We don't quite believe the speaker of the first sentence; the second speaker means nobody else loves you as much; three means yes, I really do love you; while four means the one I love is not the floozy over there but You! Just utilizing an inflection gives us all this variation, and could mean the difference between staying married or getting a divorce. We seldom realize how much the musicality of speech plays into our interpretation of words—but in oral discourse it makes all the difference. This is one reason that moving language to print becomes so difficult, for the writer must either imply the inflection through context (so that the reader hears it in her head while reading), or the writer must revert to symbols such as capitalization, underlining, italics, and exclamation marks.

Mithen, in *The Singing Neanderthals*, thinks early humans would have communicated via a system of multi-modal musical phrases without words or grammar between 1.8 and 0.25 million years ago.[9] Mithen builds his theory from one first proposed by John Blacking's in 1973, in which Blacking postulates "a prelinguistic 'musical' mode of thought and action" for early man.[10] Mithen puts this into a timeline, with "Hmmmm" (his theoretical singing/language) starting with a need for more communication due to full bipedal life (Ergaster), with "Hmmm" developing further in Erectus, and coming into fruition in the Neanderthals, who had brains the size of ours and survived in extreme hostile conditions, yet do not quite appear to have developed symbolic thought or art, at least not to the degree of Homo sapiens. Homo sapiens, Mithen believes, began segmenting the "Hmmm" phrases into words and grammar, diverging from music, some 200,000 years ago.

Our closest cousins, the common chimps and gorillas, are neither musical nor gifted in paired vocalizations; however, chimps do employ a number of vocal patterns to express emotion, such as pant hoots, pant barks, whimpers, screams, pant grunts, and copulation screams.[11] In chimps, vocalizations especially occur in times of excitement, and "dominance displays, danger vocalizations are usually spontaneous, signaling the excitement of arriving at a food source, greeting of old friends, or moments of acute fear or distress."[12] In addition, drumming is also a part of both chimp and gorilla behavior. This may even signal individuation:

> Wild chimpanzees (Pan troglodytes) generate low-frequency sounds that are audible to humans from a distance of at least 1 km away by hitting the buttresses of trees with their hands and feet. This buttress drumming occurs in discrete bouts of rapidly delivered beats that usually accompany

"pant hoots," the species-specific long-distance vocalization. Individual differences in male chimpanzee drumming were investigated during a 6-month field study in the Taï National Park, Ivory Coast. Analysis of drumming bouts recorded from six adult males revealed significant differences between individuals in three acoustic features: (1) mean duration of inter-beat interval; (2) mean number of beats per bout; and (3) mean bout duration. Preliminary analysis indicated that individuals differ in their tendency to deliver drumbeats in temporally close pairs separated by longer interbeat intervals. Qualitative examination also suggested that individuals may differ in the temporal integration of drumming into the pant hoot vocalization. These results suggest that there may be acoustic cues available for chimpanzees to recognize unseen males by their drumming performances alone. Drumming by Taï chimpanzees was also compared to drumming by chimpanzees (P.T. Schweinfurthii) from the Kanyawara study group in Kibale National Park, Uganda. The Kanyawara chimpanzees appeared to drum more often without vocalizing than did the Taï chimpanzees. When they did drum and vocalize together, the Kanyawara chimpanzees appeared to integrate their drumming later into the associated pant hoots than did the Taï chimpanzees. These results suggest the possibility that interpopulation variation exists in chimpanzee buttress drumming.[13]

Besides drumming, Jane Goodall witnessed an amazing act of communicative behavior in chimpanzees, the "rain-dance," that also involved patterned rhythmic movement, and a possible glimpse into the antecedents for music/dance/ritual. She gives this account of her experience during an interview in 2001:

One day in 1960, in the early days of my long-term study of chimpanzees, I saw something amazing. I was observing a group—seven adult males and a few females and young—on the opposite slope of a steep ravine. Suddenly, a rainstorm, which had been threatening for sometime, broke. The chimps had just finished feeding and were walking up to the open ridge. As they paused, a bolt of lightning struck, followed by a heart-stopping clap of thunder.

As if this was a signal, one of the big males stood upright and began moving rhythmically from foot to foot, eyeing the low branch of a tree. Then he charged down the slope toward the trees he had just left. There, swinging around the trunk of a small tree to break his headlong rush, he leaped into the low branches and sat motionless.

Two other males charged after him. Both broke off huge branches as they ran, dragging them and hurling them ahead. A fourth male charged, leaped into a tree, tore off a large branch, jumped with it to the ground, and ran with it down the slope. The others followed. When they reached the ridge, where the females and youngsters were watching, the males charged down again with equal vigor.

The rain fell harder. Jagged forks and brilliant flashes of lightning lit the leaden sky, and the crashing of thunder seemed to shake the very mountains. I watched, enthralled, marveling at the magnificence of these splendid beings. With a display of strength such as this, primitive man himself might have challenged the elements. Twenty minutes after it began, everything was over, and the whole group moved over the opposite ridge. I continued sitting in the rain, staring in near-disbelief at the white scars on the tree trunks and the discarded branches on the ground—all that remained to prove that the primeval rain dance had taken place at all. . . .

It is not only the rain that triggers these displays. Deep in the forest is a magnificent waterfall where one of the small, fast-flowing streams plunges some 80 feet down a sheer rock face, creating its own wind as the water is forced through a narrow fissure. Sometimes the chimpanzees, hair bristling, perform their displays in the streambed below the falls, swaying rhythmically upright, hurling rocks, climbing the slender hanging vines, and pushing out into the spray.

Afterwards a male may sit on a rock at the edge of the streams, looking up at the sheet of living water as it falls, watching as it flows past him on its way to the lake. What is he thinking? What is this thing that is always coming from above, always going away, yet always there? Is it alive?

If they had spoken language, the chimpanzees could discuss the feeling that prompted these displays. Is it something like awe? If the chimpanzee could share his feelings and questions with the others, might these wild elemental displays become ritualized into some form of animistic religion? Would they worship the falls, the deluge from the sky, the thunder and lightning—the gods of the elements? So all-powerful; so incomprehensible.[14]

Of course, some would call Goodall's interpretation of this event as "ritual" mere anthropomorphizing, a sentimental assessment of chimp behavior. But the more neuroscience tells us about our relationships to other animals, the more an over-concern for personification seems out of place. Goodall's response is no Disneyfication of nature but rather an observation of our closest living relatives reacting emotionally to incredible natural phenomena. It hardly seems a stretch to think that our common ancestors would have reacted in similar ways, and that in this kind of behavior, responding dramatically to the environment, we are indeed seeing intimations of an emotional response that leads to an "artistic" action. For the chimp behavior is not an act of survival. An act of survival would dictate, in the case of a lightning storm, getting away from the largest trees and crouching in a ditch. Neither is their behavior a mere motor action, like a shiver or a chill. Plus, there is evidence of cultural response in these displays, for it turns out "different chimpanzee groups dance with different styles. In Gombe National Park in Tanzania, the chimp rain dance is loud and frenzied. In Taï Forest National Park in the Ivory Coast, the chimpanzees dance in silent slow motion, mimicking the movements of aggression displays, like a great ape version of Tai Chi."[15] Not only can vocal acrobatics, drumming, and rhythmic dancing (all of which are essential components of music) ensue from excitement brought on by the natural environment, but bonobos, when stimulated by a new food source or feeding ground, will usually engage in communal sexual activity.[16]

MUSIC AND FOOD

In September 2001, Anne J. Blood and Robert J. Zatorre made the astounding discovery that music creates the same chemical affects as do food and sex on the brain:

> We have shown here that music recruits neural systems of reward and emotion similar to those known to respond specifically to biologically relevant stimuli, such as food and sex, and those that are artificially activated by drugs of abuse. This is quite remarkable, because music is neither strictly necessary for biological survival or reproduction, nor is it a pharmacological substance. Activation of these brain systems in response to a stimulus as abstract as music may represent an emergent property of the complexity of human cognition. Perhaps as formation of anatomical and functional links between phylogenically older, survival-related brain systems and newer, more cognitive systems increased our general capacity to assign meaning to abstract stimuli, our capacity to derive pleasure from these stimuli also increased. The ability of music to induce such intense

pleasure and its putative stimulation of endogenous reward systems suggest that, although music may not be imperative for survival of the human species, it may indeed be of significant benefit to our mental and physical well-being.[17]

But why should music have developed the same kinds of brain response as *sex and food*, both essential for survival, when music is not! Music takes time and energy, so what would have been the biological fitness benefits that would have been greater than the biological costs of putting time and energy into music? In terms of brain function, oxytocin (the social bonding chemical) is released during musical experiences (as it is in courtship, trance, and many other social interactions). Music also releases endorphins, and natural opiates used to counteract stress and pain.

To step back a minute, it's clear that I'm defining music quite loosely here, but I want to focus on one aspect of music not usually given its due: rhythm. Duke Ellington was right when he said, "It Don't Mean a Thing If It Ain't Got that Swing." Seitz, looking at the work of Swiss composer Emile Jaques-Dalcroze in light of data from neuroscience, states "that bodily processes, rhythm, and physical motion were the basis of musical expressivity and music pedagogy."[18] And as Mithen correctly points out, dance is the other element usually ignored in the discussion of music, for in most societies rhythm and dance go hand in hand. And as we all know, dancing is sexy stuff, but music might have other surprising qualities.

Michael H. Tahut, in "Rhythm, Human Temporality, and Brain Function," states that the "structured flow of time, made audible in music's temporal architecture of sound, rhythm, and polyphony, may be what excites, moves, and gives order to our feelings, thoughts and sense of movement. Music may be central to who we are." Investigators at the Max Planck Institute for Biological Cybernetics in Tübingen, Germany, scanned monkey brains while the rhesus macaques listened to either drumming or monkey calls. They found overlapping networks activated in the temporal lobe, which in humans is key to processing meaning in both speech and vision.

"Monkeys respond to drumming sounds as they would to vocalizations," researcher Christopher Kayser, a neuroscientist at the Max Planck Institute for Biological Cybernetics in Tübingen, Germany, told *LiveScience*. "Hence, drumming originated as a form of expression or communication, possibly in an ancestral species common to apes and old-world monkeys, early during primate evolution."[19] (Through YouTube videos of birds, such as Snowball, scientists have discovered that parrots can also react to rhythm and "dance" to a beat. Recent work with chimps in captivity has also shown that chimps have an affinity for music, and that they can drum to a beat, in a group setting, spontaneously creating polyrhythms.)

SEXUAL SELECTION FOR MUSIC

Sexual selection clearly seems the best answer to the question of why music began. Darwin himself believed that music must have had a direct relationship to sexual advantage in mate selection, saying that

> the impassioned orator, bard, or musician, when with his varied tones and cadences he excites the strongest emotions in his hearers, little suspects that he uses the same means by which his half-human ancestors long ago aroused each other's ardent passions, during their courtship and rivalry.[20]

Geoffrey Miller resurrects Darwin's emphasis on music and mating in "Evolution Of Human Music Through Sexual Selection":

> Consider Jimi Hendrix, for example. This rock guitarist extraordinaire died at the age of 27 in 1970, overdosing on the drugs he used to fire his musical imagination. His music output, three studio albums and hundreds of live concerts, did him no survival favours. But he did have sexual liaisons with hundreds of groupies, maintained parallel long-term relationships with at least two women, and fathered at least three children in the U.S., Germany, and Sweden. Under ancestral conditions before birth control, he would have fathered many more. Hendrix's genes for musical talent probably doubled their frequency in a single generation, through the power of attracting opposite-sex admirers. As Darwin realized, music's aesthetic and emotional power, far from indicating a transcendental origin, point to a sexual-selection origin, where too much is never enough. Our ancestral hominid-Hendrixes could never say, "OK, our music's good enough, we can stop now," because they were competing with all

the hominid-Eric-Claptons, hominid-Jerry-Garcias, and hominid-John-Lennons. The aesthetic and emotional power of music is exactly what we would expect from Sexual Selection's arms race to impress minds like ours.[21]

To anyone who has ever been involved in the music business, Miller's argument would seem so commonsensical as to not even elicit a response. But the evolutionary problem is this: If music is something that both men and women excel at, then how could it have been sexually selected? Also, if that were so, there should be some sexual dimorphism in the case of musical talent, just as there is for body size. Miller, trying to grapple with this, looked at the recording industry and discovered that males produced ten times the records as females, across all genres, with output peaking around age thirty, falling within the prime years for reproductive success. Clearly, there was something driving males, which was not driving females to the same degree. When I did an anecdotal survey of musicians I know from various genres, asking why they got into music—no matter their abilities, and some were at the very top of their professions, for the guys it was always, "To get girls." But when I asked the women it was never "To get men." Instead it was, "Because I love music," or "Because I wanted to say something with my music."

As we saw in the section on sexual selection, since human mating involves an element of female competition for males (though not to the same extent as male competition for females), musical ability in females would also have signaled *their* fitness and desirability, and we have the fact that in pair-bonding situations there is much less difference between males and females in a species on the whole. With music there is also motivation and desire within the individual. Genius has less to do with talent than obsession and desire.[22] Testosterone alone could have been responsible for igniting more of this desire for musical persistence in men.

As we will see in the trickster stories to come, there is often a tie between musicians and tricksters. Many times they are both. In this alliance, I believe we can detect a hint of the antecedents—courtship behavior—that drove our ancient ancestors to become silver-tongued devils of both song and word. For in both music and language there is the very ancient linkage to sexuality, and there is every reason to think that this is what led to the emergence of both. When most people think of "music" they think of songs, and most songs have to do with love. We crave them: listening to them on the radio going to and from work; or singing them in the shower. We wear iPods around our neck to give our lives a soundtrack. Many people associate certain songs with time periods that were important to us, as well as with particular love relationships: "That's our song." Only smell, with its most primal wiring, is more powerful for evoking emotions and memories. This explains the tendency many people have to become locked into the songs of their teen years, when hormones and emotions were running full steam. Most tend to prefer those songs and artists throughout their lifetime, whether they be Benny Goodman, Elvis, the Beatles, or The Clash.

TRIBAL SONGS OF LOVE

Songs are universal to all human societies, and they are often used to try to magically make something happen. Though there are songs for every kind of activity, love is the central pursuit. Below are examples from North American Indian and Eskimo cultures:

> *Love Song, Chippewa, North America,*
> *translated by Frances Densmore*

> A loon,
> I thought it was.
> But it was
> My love's
> Splashing oar.

> *A Woman's Song, Chippewa, North America*

> You are walking around
> Trying to remember
> What you promised
> But you can't remember

Eskimo, Dueling Song over Love, Greenland

K-
Now shall I split off words—little, sharp words
Like the wooden splinters which I hack off with my ax.
A song from ancient times—a breath of the ancestors
A song of longing—for my wife.
An impudent, black-skinned oaf has stolen her,
Has tried to belittle her.
A miserable wretch who loves human flesh—
A cannibal from famine days.
E—
Insolence that takes the breath away.
Such laughable arrogance and effrontery.
What a satirical song! Supposed to place the blame on me.
You would drive fear into my heart!
I who care not about death.
Hi! You sing about my woman who was your wench.
You weren't so loving then—she as much alone.
You forgot to prize her in song,
In stout, contest songs.
Now she is mine.
And never shall she visit singing, false lovers.
Betrayer of women in strange households.

Hummingbird Song, Tlingit, North America

> I am feeling very lonely away.
> I am singing inside.
> I am crying about myself.

8

ETHICS

When I do good, I feel good; when I do bad, I feel bad. That's my religion.

—Abraham Lincoln

For all animal life there must be a system of value—even for single-celled organisms. Motion itself is related to value and is the primary reason we have a brain—to direct us toward good or bad—toward that which will keep us healthy and away from that which will do us harm. The complexity of *how* values are assessed, of course, accelerates in creatures with the development of a central nervous system and brain. When we arrive at social animals, and eventually ourselves, the notion of value becomes multi-dimensional, no longer just a matter of movement for the individual, but the organism must take into consideration the regulation of actions affecting the political concerns of an entire society of other individuals of which it is a part. As we shall see when examining the trickster stories, at heart this is what they explore: how should one behave amongst a world of others.

From the time of the first myth, we humans have speculated as to our condition, asking, "Who are we, and why do we do what we do?" Implied in those questions is this one: "How are we are *supposed* to act?" In tribal society the myths themselves present these dilemmas in a covert and literary fashion, and "laws" for behavior are not expressed formally. With the advent of state-level society, writing led to the codification of behavior in laws transcribed into stone (instead of being just loose and unspecified societal norms), such as the Code of Ur-Nammu, king of Ur (ca. 2050 BC), the Laws of Eshnunna (ca. 1930 BC) the codex of Lipit-Ishtar of Isin (ca. 1870 BC), the Code of Hammurabi (1760 BC), as well as others. The later Jewish Mosiac Code is the one most of us know as the Ten Commandments. Number seven of the Code of Hammurabi serves as an example of these legal proclamations: "If any one buy from the son or the slave of another man, without witnesses or a contract, silver or gold, a male or female slave, an ox or a sheep, an ass or anything, or if he take it in charge, he is considered a thief and shall be put to death."[1] The societies that developed these laws were theocracies—church and state aligned—so that the ultimate authority was seen as having come from the gods—and through the gods to their divine emissaries on earth—the sons of gods—the monarchs. Western tradition saw this as part of the "natural order" in that these laws (in Christian and Jewish tradition—the Mosiac) derived from the very gods who created the natural world.

However, such laws were also seen as reasonable (whether the antecedent for them be divine or mortal), in that they kept order and maintained fairness in the sense that a legal precedent was established that theoretically would apply to all for whom justice must be administered. Aristotle wrote that human happiness depended upon reason and that to be virtuous was a logical result of a reasoned (logos) life.

Following Aristotle in Western tradition, "reason" became the primary assumptive force for calculating ethical value; therefore, philosophers have worked diligently to create prescriptions for morality under the assumption that reasonable people will adhere to reasonable arguments and act accordingly. Reason became that element within us that could vanquish our animal nature, taming us into submission so *societies* of rational order might follow. Reason, as a creation of the gods, was also natural, as humans were endowed with this property.

I will come back to address aspects of Aristotelian ethics, but first I would like to turn to Thomas Hobbes (1651), the first to really challenge the Aristotelian view, for Hobbes saw human beings as both amoral and asocial, and perceived that values were either "natural" or "artificial," and the two were cataclysmically separate. Hobbes took umbrage with the idea that nature provided any kind of moral foundation. There was nothing naturally good in nature that could constitute a system for human morality. Hobbes believed that it was only in the world of artifice that mankind could succeed, for the world of nature would lead to chaotic despotism, ignorance, and danger, with "no knowledge of the face of the earth; no account of time; no arts; no letters; no society; continual fear, and danger of violent death; and the life of man, solitary, poor, nasty, brutish, and short."[2] As James Rachels explains Hobbes's position,

> to escape the state of nature, then, people must agree to the establishment of rules to govern their relations with one another, and they must agree to the establishment of an agency—the state—with the power necessary to enforce those rules. . . . This agreement is called the *social contract*.[3]

John Locke's (1632–1704) political theory was founded in opposition to Hobbes, for Locke saw reason and tolerance as attributes of human nature, though like Hobbes, Locke also saw selfishness as an essential human trait, from which he developed the supply and demand theory of economic structure. Locke also believed that when born, the human mind was a "tabula rasa," a blank slate. Ethical Egoism, the belief that society runs best by the fulfillment of each individual's personal desires, is also linked to Locke—a system that has become the bedrock of capitalistic belief as articulated in Adam Smith's *The Wealth of Nations* (1776), where he states than an "invisible hand" guides an economic policy based on personal greed that will maintain a perfect equilibrium. The term *laissez-faire* has often been used in association with this position, one which admonishes the deregulation of the private sector while abhorring any governmental incursion into the economy for the "public" good (as good in this sense is always seen as private). Humans were reasonable actors, who when acting reasonably (in their own interests) would create societies that would approach reasonable perfection.

In Western tradition, another important philosophical position is the deontological argument initiated by Immanuel Kant (1724–1804). This position states that mankind needs rules by which to live (in close relationship to social contract theory), with the caveat being that those rules should be followed under all circumstances. Rules, in Kant's philosophy, do not depend upon religious decree; they stem from reason alone. As James Rachels says of Kant's philosophy, "The only way moral goodness can exist is for rational creatures to apprehend what they should do and, acting from a sense of duty, do it. . . . Thus if there were no rational beings, the moral dimension of the world would simply disappear."[4]

Utilitarianism, the other major Western philosophical argument (from the name of a book written by John Mill in 1861) advocates the moral position that in any circumstance the correct form of action is the one that leads to the greater good for the greater number of people, once again a prescriptive position based on reason: "According to the Greatest Happiness Principle . . . the ultimate end, with reference to and for the sake of which all other things are desirable (whether we are considering our own good or that of other people), is an existence exempt as free as possible from pain, and as rich as possible in enjoyments."[5] Interestingly enough, Mill advances that moral decisions based upon Utilitarian principles should also extend to "the whole of sentient creation" (Rachels), a position that the West has never seriously considered.

THE FALLACY OF THE NATURALISTIC FALLACY: IS-OUGHT

Scottish philosopher David Hume (1711–1776) was secular in his thinking and demanded empirical evidence in the determination of truth. Yet, he realized that inductive reasoning, making inferences based upon observable data, was not reliable. Just because we perceive constancy in nature, one could not logically infer that such would be the case once you took your eyes off of the subject at hand. It is "consistent and conceivable" that nature would change. Instead of reason being the dominant power that allows us to make determinations of constancy, Hume postulated that it was natural instinct that allowed us to make inductive inferences, stating that "the lives of men depend upon the same laws as the lives of all other animals."[6] It is our animal nature that allows us to proceed in the world and to make the necessary decisions for survival, and that allows for reason itself: "Reason is, and ought only to be the slave of the passions, and can never pretend to any other office than to serve and obey them."[7] Morality then, in Hume's estimation depends primarily upon emotion, and does not derive from logic: "Morals excite passions, and produce or prevent actions. Reason itself is utterly impotent in this particular. The rules of morality, therefore, are not conclusions of our reason."[8]

Hume's interpretation is strikingly similar to what neuroscientist Antonio Damasio has shown in his research—that there is no such thing as pure logic devoid of emotion. Yet, ironically, another of Hume's advances, which has become known as Hume's law, seems to say the opposite. From the Stanford Encyclopedia of Philosophy:

> Hume famously closes the section of the Treatise that argues against moral rationalism by observing that other systems of moral philosophy, proceeding in the ordinary way of reasoning, at some point make an unremarked transition from premises linked only by "is" to propositions linked by "ought" (expressing a new relation)—a deduction that seems to Hume "altogether inconceivable" (T3.1.1.27). Attention to this transition would "subvert all the vulgar systems of morality, and let us see, that the distinction of vice and virtue is not founded merely on the relations of objects, nor is perceiv'd by reason."[9]

The Is-Ought argument is usually assumed to mean that regarding ethical judgments, nothing that occurs in nature can be assumed to be prescriptive regarding how one *ought* to behave. This essentially harkens back to Hobbes—the notion that nature is brutish and offers no template for human ethics—hence the term Naturalistic Fallacy. But this interpretation contradicts Hume's entire thesis: that ethics are not derived from reason but are emotive. Hume answers the one question that those who continue to believe in the Naturalist Fallacy fail to see: From whence did "ought" arrive? (This is especially true in light of the fact that we find the same basic repetition of human moral codes throughout our species—which I will return to in the discussion on cultural relativism). As Larry Arnhart states in *Darwinian Natural Right,*

> If we accept the common view of Hume as having argued that we cannot infer what ought to be from what is the case, then it would seem that he contradicts himself by deriving moralit from the natural inclinations of human beings. The contradiction disappears, however, once we see

that the dichotomy between is and ought falsely attributed to Hume was actually first formulated by Immanuel Kant, who used it as an argument against the kind of ethical naturalism developed by Hume! Furthermore, once this point is understood, it becomes clear that while the proponents of Darwinian naturalism are Humeans, their critics are Kantians.[10]

As Arnhart states, "Kant's separation of is and ought treats morality as an autonomous realm of human experience governed by its own internal logic with no reference to anything in human nature such as natural desires or nature."[11] Darwin saw that instead of there existing a dualism between nature and ethics, the entire realm of emotions which derive from the fact of social interactions between animals of the same species constitutes the very basis of moral being:

> It has, I think, now been shewn that man and the higher animals, especially the Primates, have some few instincts in common. All have the same senses, intuitions, and sensations—similar passions, affections, and emotions, even the more complex ones, such as jealousy, suspicion, emulation, gratitude, and magnanimity; they practise deceit and are revengeful; they are sometimes susceptible to ridicule, and even have a sense of humour; they feel wonder and curiosity; they possess the same faculties of imitation, attention, deliberation, choice, memory, imagination, the association of ideas, and reason, though in very different degrees. The individuals of the same species graduate in intellect from absolute imbecility to high excellence. They are also liable to insanity, though far less often than in the case of man.[12]

This brings us back to Aristotle, who derived his system of ethics from biology. He said, "Thought by itself moves nothing," and that choice involves "desiring reason" or "reasoning desire." Aristotle saw that politics (social attachment and construct) was a natural part of human behavior, and in the root of this natural political desire, stemming from biology, arose moral sensibility. His Virtue ethics are based on the proposition that any prescriptive system of ethical rules will always fail, as ethical behavior, rooted in biology, is always a complicated matter involving a multiplicity of instincts, as well as cultural and historical influences and concerns. In other words, goodness can never be determined by a Deontological or Universalist argument, both of which are simplistic in design and impossible in application. To say one should not kill is meaningless when someone is coming at you with a knife and it's you or him. Likewise, the Social Contract theory, based on rules, is meaningless without some basic social sense imbued in the species in the first place. We could never have enough law enforcement officers to control the population, and then again they'd all be corrupt and in need of supervision themselves.

Darwin believed that it was in the realm of attachment between parents and offspring that feelings of empathy and "love" arose in various species, and that these served as the backbone for the further development of human emotions that led to a more highly refined sensibility of ethical behavior. This is exactly what Aristotle believed nearly 2500 years earlier: that the prolonged requirement for parental care is what led to social love and it was precisely the same sentiment described by Hume: "that the natural moral sentiments that bind people in families can expand to embrace larger groups."[13] Of course, none of these thinkers knew anything of genes, but as Robert Wright says in *The Moral Animal*, they play an essential part in the story:

> Genes don't magically sense the presence of copies of themselves in other organisms and try to save them. [Here discussing kinship theory of reciprocity]. Genes aren't clairvoyant, or even conscious; they don't "try" to do anything. But should a gene appear that happens to make its vehicle behave in ways that help the survival or reproduction prospects of other vehicles likely to contain a copy of that gene, then the gene may thrive, even if prospects for its vehicle are lowered in the process. . . . This logic could apply, as in this case, to a gene that inclines a mammal to produce a warning call when it sees a threat to its home burrow, where relatives reside. The logic could also apply to a gene that leads an insect to be sterile, so long as the insect spends its life helping fertile relatives. . . . [and to genes that help humans] sense early on who their siblings are and thereafter share food with them, give guidance to them, defend them, and so on—genes, in other words, leading to sympathy, empathy, compassion: genes for love.[14]

The fallacy of the Naturalistic Fallacy is quite apparent in lieu of the past twenty years of the Darwinian renaissance in all aspects of science, which has revolutionized our approach to answering the oldest questions we have about ourselves. Whereas the entire tradition of philosophy has been purely speculative, with the advent of neuroscience we finally have tools available that can scientifically answer some of the most perplexing questions of our species that philosophy had previously tried to address. Now we have a vast amount of technological resources, such as MRI scans, DNA research, and more, yielding empirical evidence, which shows many of the old answers to have been wrong. More has been gleaned about the nature of the human brain in the last ten years than in all previous time. For this reason, scientists such as E. O. Wilson have been calling for the coming together of Science, Philosophy, and Ethics:

> For much of this century, moral philosophy has been constrained by the supposed absolute gap between is and ought, and the consequent belief that the facts of life cannot of themselves yield an ethical blueprint for future action. For this reason, ethics has sustained an eerie existence largely apart from Science. Its most respected interpreters still believe that reasoning about right and wrong can be successful without a knowledge of the brain, the human organ where all the decisions about right and wrong are made. Ethical premises are typically treated in the manner of mathematical propositions: directives supposedly independent of human evolution, with a claim to ideal, eternal truths.
>
> While many substantial gains have been made in our understanding of the nature of moral thought and action, insufficient use has been made of knowledge of the brain and its evolution. Beliefs in extrasomatic moral truths and in an absolute is/ought barrier are wrong. Moral premises relate only to our physical nature and are the result of an idiosyncratic genetic history—a history which is nevertheless powerful and general enough within the human species to form working codes. The time has come to turn moral philosophy into an applied Science because, as the geneticist Hermann J. Muller urged in 1959, 100 years without Darwin are enough.[15]

FAIRNESS AND JUSTICE IN THE ANIMAL WORLD

Trickster stories, in which taboos are constantly broken, can only exist if there are rules in place before Trickster has arrived (and keep in mind—Trickster is usually a god). The very fact Trickster exists as a universal phenomenon, as a character who deals with moral concerns, goes to prove that our human sense of morality is, at base, extremely similar across the globe. Actions that mitigate toward justice can only occur if something in the brain is wired for fair play. What may be a surprise to some is the fact that we humans are not the only animals who have compassion, empathy, and social codes of behavior.

Besides having social codes, animals by nature also exhibit protean behavior, meaning they are flexible and can do the unexpected (this is an important aspect that defines Trickster). Animals can make unpredictable choices, which often are the very choices that allow them to escape predation or find food. Choice is inherent in the notion of fairness. Justice can only develop in a behavioral system that allows for different kinds of actions. Of course choice is not unlimited (Darwin saw right away that his theory of evolution was problematic for free will) but choice at some level defines what it is to be an animal—to go here or go there. Some of these choices for higher animals involve the behavior of affection and courteous treatment of others. Of course in social animals, like primates, with mirror cells and awareness of others' intentions, an individual's behavioral choices often determine his or her rank in society. To survive, one needs friends.

There are numerous examples of animals exhibiting "caring behavior" within their own species, and there are cases even of such between species. Marc Bekoff, a biologist who studies emotions in animals, relates cases such as these: a troop of a 100 rhesus monkeys in India that brought "traffic to a halt after a baby monkey was hit by a car":

> A teenage female elephant nursing an injured leg is knocked over by a rambunctious hormone-laden teenage male. An older female sees this happen, chases the male away, and goes back to the younger female and touches her sore leg with her trunk.
>
> Eleven elephants rescue a group of captive antelope in KwaZula-Natal; the matriarch elephant undoes all of the latches on the gates of the enclosure with her trunk and lets the gate swing open so the antelope can escape.
>
> A rat in a cage refuses to push a lever for food when it sees that another rat receives an electric shock as a result. A male Diana monkey who learned to insert a token into a slot to obtain food helps a female who can't get the hang of the trick, inserting the token for her and allowing her to eat the food reward.[16]

Anyone who has ever owned two or more dogs knows that perceptions of fairness play a huge part in their social interactions. This concept of fairness has been found to exist in a number of species:

> Imagine the following situation. Nancy loves cucumbers, and will always eat them if given an opportunity. However, one day she sees Winnie getting a grape (which they both like better than cucumbers) and then she is only given a cucumber! Nancy immediately throws the cucumber on the ground and turns away. Does this sound like anyone you know? Substitute chocolate for vegetables and the answer is probably yes. However, Nancy and Winnie are both capuchin monkeys showing a species normal response to distributional inequity (Brosnan and de Waal, 2003a). Capuchin monkeys are not the only ones who react to inequity, either. Chimpanzees throw temper tantrums if their expectations are violated. Social canids (e.g. wolves, coyotes, and domestic dogs) have a set of social rules regarding how rough play among juveniles can be, and if these rules are violated, the offending individual is excluded from play sessions. These are only a few examples in a relatively new field of study, but even from these it seems that animals do react when they feel that they have been treated inequitably.[17]

Social justice in species has a correlation to order, and order with status/hierarchy, which itself stems from the struggles over mating and food preferences, the dominant aspects of animal's lives.

In one of the most astounding studies of primate behavior ever, neurobiologist Robert Sapolsky made an incredible discovery about aggression when studying stress in the lives of olive baboons. Sapolsky found that hierarchy and stress have an exact correlation, with those at the bottom experiencing most stress, leading to severely adverse health. The male baboons at the top are virtually free of stress—but they are aggressive bullies, sadistic, and antagonistic to others below their rank. In the troop Sapolsky was studying there was a bizarre occurrence in which the high-ranking males were all killed after accidentally eating some poison. To Sapolsky's astonishment, the troop continued on without them but with a complete change in behavior. The aggression and bullying ended with the death of the most dominant males, and a new way of being baboon for the troop came into being, that has continued now for decades, even after other male baboons from different troops moved in. This study shows clearly that different ways of establishing hierarchy can emerge in primates through a shift in group dynamics, and that elements of culture can arise that can continue to ameliorate brutal male behavior.[18]

Studies by Caroline Zink have shown that hierarchy is wired into the human brain just as it is in other primates/mammals, and most species. In humans one's status is constantly being calculated against that of others. As Zink says, hierarchy is "influential in everything we do, whether it's boss-employee, teacher-student, coach-athlete."[19] Three brain regions appear to be involved in the establishment of hierarchical status:

> the anterior cingulate, an area that has been shown to monitor conflict and resolve discrepancies; the medial prefrontal cortex, which processes thoughts about other people; and the precuneus, a newly discovered region that some scientists think may be the seat of self-consciousness, the brain's ability to think about itself.[20]

Recent studies in envy have also corroborated the brain's pre-wired ability to react to hierarchical social conditions:

> Now researchers are gleaning insights into the neural and evolutionary underpinnings of envy, and why it can feel like a bodily illness or a physical blow. They're also tracing the pathway of envy's equally petty foil, the sensation of schadenfreude—taking pleasure when those whom you envied are themselves brought down low.
>
> Reporting in the current issue of the journal *Science*, researchers at the National Institute of Radiological Sciences in Japan and their colleagues described brain-scanning studies of subjects who were told to imagine themselves as protagonists in social dramas with characters of greater or lesser status or achievement. When confronting characters that the participants admitted to envying, brain regions involved in registering physical pain were aroused: the higher the subjects rated their envy, the more vigorously flared the pain nodes in the brain's dorsal anterior cingulate cortex and related areas.
>
> Conversely, the researchers said, when subjects were given a chance to imagine the golden one's downfall, the brain's reward circuits were activated, again in proportion to the strength of envy's sting: the subjects who felt the greatest envy the first time around reacted to news of their rival's

misfortune with a comparatively livelier response in the dopamine-rich pleasure centers of, for example, the ventral striatum. "We have a saying in Japanese, 'The misfortunes of others are the taste of honey,'" said Hidehiko Takahashi, the first author on the report. "The ventral striatum is processing that 'honey.'"[21]

That our trickster brains have been programmed through evolution to detect fairness and unfairness should not be a surprise, as one's being depends upon correctly interpreting one's place within the greater social network and negotiating one's status through a maze of relationships; in the end this has everything to do with determining if an organism's genes will live or die. Life in a group has tremendous benefits (one-celled organisms pairing up into two-celled, then many-celled organisms, began this process billions of years ago), yet there are also tremendous stresses. Trickster stories portray these conflicts of hierarchy and status, fairness and deceit, as well as the emotions of envy and jealousy, lust, and hate. In the stories, we often see both the egalitarian/democratic spirit and the feudal/monarchial one, sometimes existing side by side. Both are represented in our group politics and both stem from the very structures of our brains. The themes in trickster stories tell of a moral code, shaped by culture to be sure, but essentially universal and innate. The trickster stories, just as in the story about the baboons, also show that we primates are capable of acting in a variety of ways, with "ethical" behavior a part of who we are.

(9)

STORYTELLING AND THE
THEORY OF MIND

If you don't know the trees you may be lost in the forest, but if you don't know the stories you may be lost in life.

—Siberian Elder

Storytelling involves an array of mental activity—the aural construction and reception of sound symbols, rich with connotation and association, as metaphors and schemas rise, blend, fall, while momentary elements of narration are held in working memory and then reinterpreted by the new information that follows—since stories are necessarily linked to time. While all this is going on, our brains are continually reassessing the entire narrative past, while anticipating the future course of narrative events. And on top of all this, the story, as we listen, is making us feel something—fearful, happy, sad, shocked, sexually awakened, jealous, worried, or embarrassed—as the memories of our own lived experiences come flooding through. For each of us visualizes the details and interprets the meaning of stories through his or her own subjective past. If the protagonist is scared we're a little scared ourselves. If the main character is sitting on top of the world, we are also a little bit inflated. We feel stories because of our lived past and our emotional memories.

In the first breath of the story we hear that the wolf is stealing from the forest. In the second utterance, we learn he is hungry. In the third, we learn the wolf is hungry for *us*. Our connective mind snaps the pieces together and works them into a present whole, as we listen logically, putting two and two together, but listening emotionally as well, as our hearts race and our palms sweat, as our attention is focused on the teller from whom we want to find out what will happen next. Emotion and feeling are at the heart of stories and are what give stories value. We *care* what happens next. Story is an activity we never tire of, for it is the way the human mind works. As P. C. Hogan says, stories are universal:

> Literature—or, more properly, verbal art—is not produced by nations, periods, and so on. It is produced by people. And these people are incomparably more alike than not. They share ideas, perceptions, desires, aspirations, and—what is most important for our purposes—emotions. Verbal art certainly has national, historical, and other inflections. The study of such particularity is tremendously important. However, literature is by all people at all times. As Paul Kiparsky put it, "literature is neither recent nor a historical invention. In fact no human community lacks a literature"; no group is "so wretched that it does not express its memories and desires in stories and poems."[1]

We put the pieces of experience together every day—trying to figure out the world and our place in it—through both the large stories and the small, both subconsciously (95 percent or more) and with consciousness. Language allows both the creation of new worlds and the ability for us to move into that territory through imagination, taking us out of numbing drudgery and giving us freedom. Gossip was one such freedom that language allowed—further connecting our web of human relationships and infusing those connections with theater (drama and comedy). There were many more freedoms language allowed us—mythic worlds, time, calendars, rituals, religion, even hope itself. Language carved up the world into not only more explicit divisions than pre-language categories and thought schemas could: me and you, you and him, them and us. Language also divided the world into taxonomies: the tusked, the hooved, the winged. It was no accident that the first task God gave man in the Garden of Eden was to name the animals, for with naming comes differentiation and power through defined networks and an explication of relationship: kinship, lineages, family trees (not only between humans and other humans, but between humans and animals, as well as animals and animals, plants and plants). Patricia S. Churchland has called the brain's ability to parse the world, "cognitive compression," which "helps to categorize the world and reduce the complexity of conceptual structures to a manageable scale."[2] Language allows for the natural categorizing process of brain activity (which creates a mapped version of the world) to be cast it into an exterior communicative web. A portion of an individual's mapped mind can be shared through the oral transference of story.

UNCONSCIOUSNESS AND CONSCIOUSNESS

The mapping mind is directly related to the greatest mystery of all: that of consciousness. As John Horgan says in "Can Science Explain Consciousness?"

> Investigators are probing its [the brain's] deepest recesses with increasingly powerful tools, ranging from microelectrodes, which can discern the squeaks of individual neurons, to magnetic resonance imaging and positron emission tomography, which can amplify the cortical symphony . . . [which has allowed] "a growing number of scientists" to look into questions regarding "the most elusive and inescapable of all phenomena: consciousness, our immediate, subjective awareness of the world and ourselves."[3]

The problem of consciousness is being examined from many angles, and there are numerous findings, many of which are converging. David J. Chalmers says in "The Puzzle of Conscious Experience," "consciousness is subjective, so there is no way to monitor it in others. But this difficulty is an obstacle, not a dead end. For a start, each one of us has access to our own experiences, a rich trove that can be used to formulate theories."[4] Those experiences are turned into stories, as our minds naturally create narratives, the most important perhaps being the narrative each of us has about ourselves. We naturally create a mythic "me," which is nearly always imagined as a traveler on a journey, as we live in the arrow of time. As we progress on our path, we both collect anecdotes and attempt to make sense of them. While the right side of the brain primarily deals with collecting information, the left side handles making sense of the information that has been collected, creating the stories that form our lives.[5] Kotre describes these two aspects of the brain, which Sedonie A. Smith in turn calls the "librarian element" and the "mythmaking element."[6] The mythmaking element is the creation of the "self," that autobiographical sense born from bits and pieces of memory and turned into the perceptions of "this is who I am," projecting the feeling of a single being who, though constantly changing through time, remains somehow the same.

But memory is not what most people believe—a video tape in the brain that plays back the past. Instead, memory is something that is reconstituted continually *in the present*. The brain forms connections with each moment that is memorized, which involves emotion, images, sounds, smells, and context. At the moment of remembering it reassembles these elements, igniting the same sensory elements throughout the brain as in the moment the memory first occurred. Antonio Damasio's latest hypothesis is that memory is retained through a combination of the disposition and the mapping systems of the brain. Neurons control movement, something that plants did not evolve. Neurons can also create maps of the body and of the outside world that the body lives in. Mapmaking is the primary function of an advanced brain. A "slice" of neurons operates the way a pixilated screen does: certain molecules in the brain are turned off or on to replicate the world the eye takes in, just as certain pixels are activated or are inactive on the pixilated screen. A computer screen can be made to look like anything—an old black and white movie, a luscious tropical plant, an African lion, even the world itself spinning blue and white in outer space. The pixels that constitute the screen can activate instantly, revealing an unlimited number of patterns. Neurons also mimic on a grid formed from what the senses see, hear, feel, taste, touch, all of which Damasio calls images. By mapping, the brain literally replicates what it takes in from the world, later translating these images into meaning. An apple, for instance would be portrayed as oval shaped, red, shiny on a visual grid. But the brain/mind translates that different ways, depending upon the larger context. This brings us to another essential part of mapping: the creating of categories. The brain allows for a system of value—a hierarchy of levels. Food is elementary, but there are more complex meanings that fall under an element of an apple. It exists in relation to all the other apple pieces that are part of the category it "lives" in, such as an apple falling from a tree hitting Newton on the head, or an apple under a tree in which two naked humans stand. Immediately, we grasp a higher order of meaning, for the apple will remind us of sin and sexuality—the Garden of Eden—and categories of religion, ethics, morality, and many more, will be opened up. The wiring we are born with, and the wiring we acquire from experience both work to interpret "apple" and all of its various meanings and manifestations.

The brain takes in data from the senses and arranges it into categories to create order out of chaos. It does this for reasons of survival. Imagine a *Homo erectus* looking out on an African landscape. She would have to make sense of colors and shapes: a herd of elephants, a volcano, three lionesses, two thousand zebra, a river of crocodiles, and a fierce wind. The brain evolved as a way of assessing values in order to make predictions about the future and how a particular story might end up depending upon the actions one might take. Any of those things in the landscape just mentioned could be a threat. The lions are large dangerous animals, but they also have respectable brains and are probably in fear of the volcano that is spouting ash and not much in the mood for a meal. The crocs, less brainy, probably have little awareness of the volcano and would gulp you right up, so you have to worry about them. The elephants are smart but very aware and more dangerous even than lions (more people are killed by elephants in Africa than lions) as they could stampede, like the zebras could, who are less intelligent, but there are more of them. One *might* be able get out of the way of these large creatures by observing them closely and climbing into the trees at the right time. But then again the volcano spew could be very dangerous, full of chemicals that could hurt lung tissue or even cause death if inhaled, which the wind will carry, also fanning fires. So the best path would probably be to not go the way the wind is blowing, but go at right angles from the wind, or to get behind it on the other side of the volcano. The brain would have instantly put things in categories to make such an assessment of these threats: animals and non-animals; predators and stampeding animals; wind and volcano smoke.

But mapping, and creating categories are not the only things the neurons allow. The older job they had was in creating dispositions (the ability to learn to go this way instead of that way when a particular stimulus

occured). The dispositional system is ancient, the one primitive creatures use to make decisions that initiate action. A stimulus occurs and a
muscle reacts in a particular way. Dispositions are simple and effective.
The mapping system is much more sophisticated and recent, allowing
for greater precision and greater predictive power. But when the mapping system evolved, the disposition system did not go away. According
to Damasio, the two united as a way of saving space. Maps are costly
in terms of space as they take up a lot of "memory." Damasio believes
that the disposition system encodes mapmaking, making more mental
space available. When a memory is being recalled, the dispositional system (like a computer program that encrypts a large file and reduces it
for storage or transmission) contains a formula to reconstitute the map.
The map recharges the molecules in the sensory cortices—as they were
excited originally—recreating the senses, context, mood, and ambience
of the original moment and merging these with what is going on at the
moment a memory is being recalled. According to Damasio:

> *the disposition was commanding the process of reactivating and putting*
> *together aspects of past perception*, wherever they had been processed
> and then locally recorded. Specifically, the dispositions would act on a
> host of early sensory cortices originally engaged by perception. The dispo-
> sitions would do so by dint of connections diverging from the disposition
> site back to early sensory cortices. In the end, the locus where memory
> records would actually be played back would not be that different from
> the locus of original perception.[7]

You sit in your chair and think of a candy store you went to one day as
a kid. The dispositional part of the brain connects with the mapmaking
part, and the old map comes back, igniting the original sensory areas
of the brain as they were in their original time zone. It's like you can
taste your favorite chocolate bar all over again, and be dazzled by all the
candy packages and wrappers everywhere; you see the woman working
the counter with her bright red lipstick and smell her perfume, and you
are reminded of your mom telling you to quit going into the candy store
every day or else you'll get fat. You remember all that and much more
tied to that era, while at the same time your memory is tied to the present, to the fact that you are sitting in a chair now, twenty years later,
twenty pounds fatter than you were in middle school. So you feel guilty

about that and tell yourself that you'll go on a diet, but first you need one more chocolate bar, so you get up and go out the door and drive to the nearest place that sells candy bars, while all the time you can still hear your mom's voice in your head telling you not to do it.

Of course, memories are imperfect, not *exact* representations, and our interpretations of events from the past is subject to contemporary biases. And all of this activity is being processed in the subconscious. What "the brain computes," Michael Gazzaniga states, in *The Mind's Past*, the mind is the "last to know." The conscious mind is at the very end of the line in terms of events. The "interpreter" part of the brain "reconstructs the brain events and in doing so makes telling errors of perception, memory, and judgment." For this reason, Gazzaniga states flatly that "biography is fiction," and that "autobiography is hopelessly inventive."[8] The literature regarding false memory is voluminous, from episodes of induced "memory" of psychotherapy "revealing" mythical childhood sexual molestations to the well-known unreliability of first-hand witnesses in court. Studies of those who have had their corpus callosum severed (the connecting nerves that hold together the left and right hemispheres of the brain) show repeatedly that in such patients the left brain invents stories to explain what the right brain is doing.

From an evolutionary point of view, it makes sense that higher-brained animals would have developed a *fairly* reliable memory, for it is an essential tool for survival: the ability to recall environments that offer food, shelter, water; the ability to remember one's friends and en-emies within a social environment in which alliances play a crucial role; the ability to remember the lessons of behavior that might engender survival, such as the right food choices, the right way to avoid preda-tors, and the most successful mating strategies. Evidence has shown that memories with greater image detail are more reliable—so a water-ing hole by two palms next to a mountain that looks like a pyramid—is probably a more factual memory than the piece of gossip someone told you at the bar six weeks ago about their sister. Memory about people and events can be very unreliable, which is why first-person testimony in criminal cases is notoriously bad (and why many innocent people are locked up in jail). Memories are creations of the "self."

That "self," created by the brain, the protagonist "me," "I," is neither learned nor taught but is universal to human experience. Its centrality to our being must also have served some evolutionary purpose, for unlike other higher animals—who hold an immediate sense of core consciousness with memory of past events, locations, and relationships—there is no evidence that even our closest cousins, chimps and gorillas, contain within their minds an autobiographical self, at least not to the degree we do (chimps, dolphins, elephants, magpies, and some other animals can *recognize themselves*, through experiments involving self identification in a mirror, but that is not the same).

Damasio makes clear that the "self" is constituted from all the cells and organs of the body, the organs and primitive brain areas that the brain maps. The self is not something derived just from higher consciousness. But what advantages might the constructed self have had for our ancestors, when there's plenty of evidence that it is not always reliable? Is it just an accidental by-product of having a large brain and greater intelligence, just an auxiliary to consciousness? Or is it an accident of language development—that once we began to talk we automatically began to practice self-talk—that incessant chattering of the mind that we all experience daily—which bolstered an already dormant mythical story-telling talent (tied to basic cause and effect processing of schema manufacturing) creating the story of self? Bickle points out that the wiring of self-talk (from studies of brain activity through scanning) has very little to do with cognitive ability:

> Given the limited access enjoyed by the language regions to neural networks that subserve specific cognitive and behavioral tasks, these narratives are actually outright fabrications, as is the self-in-control they create and express. The linguistic contents of these inner narratives about the self's causal control are false; the causal effects they attribute to deliberations and exhortations are pieces of fiction that don't square with the known anatomical and biological facts. Cognitive processing is occurring throughout the cortex (and subcortically). But activity in the brain's language regions, and hence the neurally realized narrative self, neither accurately reflects *nor causally affects* very much of what is going on [emphasis his].[9]

Yet, regardless of the unreliability of self-talk and the lack of empirical validity of self-narrative, we find the stories we make up essential to the concept of "me." While every living thing (from the gene on) has an innate and tenacious desire to live, for large-brained Homo sapiens, the story of oneself (and one's tribe), is probably—outside of the individual drive for hierarchical dominance and reproduction—the greatest human obsession. I think the two are intricately linked. Having a self gives purpose and drive to the individual that could very well have an adaptive quality for survival, spurring an individual to want to keep going in even the most desperate circumstances. In order to make sense from an evolutionary perspective it would have to have had some survival ability for an individual, even though sense of self is also tied to the tribe's mythic system of belief and most elements of culture. Possibly, a sense of self could be caused by mirror cells and social awareness. However it came into being, self becomes a driving force,. As the genes desire immortality through reproduction, so do our embodied minds want to reach immortality through stories that live on after our bodies rot. The inscribed gravestone in the local cemetery is such a testament, as is the Pyramid of Giza, and the terracotta warriors of China. Having dominion over the earth essentially means imprinting one's particular story upon the environment. As a species, we have gone to war over and over again to make sure that *our* stories and not someone else's are the ones that live on. In a sense, story is the cultural equivalent of the gene, and to have a story (for an individual or a group) has often meant fighting tooth and nail to insure it's not forgotten. Story is the encapsulation of the entire imagined identity—from past, to present, and future—and the drive to preserve the "self" of the individual or the tribe is a powerful force.

W. J. Freeman calls the human ability to create and interpret stories of self *"the examined life"* and he makes the point that the "truth" of events can often only be ascertained beyond the moment in which they occur—just as we finish reading a story and look back upon the earlier episodes with a new clarity of what the preceding events mean.[10] Freeman says that this ability is valuable to the human condition, giving us greater insight into the meaning of our lives. But it still would have to be the consequence of natural or sexual selection.

THEORY OF MIND

Throughout the animal kingdom, it is social animals who test highest on intelligence tests (of course, we humans are the ones defining "intelligence").

And a general consensus is emerging that high intelligence stems from individuals within a species interacting with their peers, where knowledge of others within the group is required for survival. For example, in primates one's relationship to others must constantly be calculated to establish and secure one's place in society. A primate must know its rank in relationship to others—including a history of interactions—and be able to be cognizant of numerous individuals. For humans, Theory of Mind, knowing the minds of others goes to the heart of our humanity, and we have this ability in spades. We *must* be able to inhabit the world of another through imagination. We see people around us and believe we know how they think and feel. We can even imagine what another person knows and feels about someone else's knowing and feeling of yet another person far away. We can conjure up, and store, multiple scenarios in our minds, mapping all these varied perspectives at once. And in our species, children are able to understand what other people think at about the age of four. They begin to anticipate another person's consciousness and perspective and include it in their own.

A 1978 article by psychologists David Premack and Guy Woodruff, "Does the Chimpanzee Have a 'Theory of Mind,'" began the scientific look at how we think about others. While scientists still argue to what degree non-human animals possesses a Theory of Mind, there is no doubt that human beings are the masters of the skill. As Jesse Bering says in *The Belief Instinct*, having a Theory of Mind "was so useful for our ancestors in explaining and predicting other people's behaviors that it has completely flooded our evolved social brains."[11] In other words, we continually construe the intent of others (while we also *imagine* intent in forces of nature, inanimate objects, animals (even attributing natural acts as emanating from the gods). Even if we don't get it right all the time, the fact that we can accurately predict the behavior of other humans most of the time gave enough advantage to our ancestors so that the Theory of Mind trait is now part of our genetic endowment.

Storytelling is really Theory of Mind fictionalized, for each and every story deals with the psychology of intent: what drives a character, and how will those forces influence a character to behave. In story, we try to coax out the elements of motivation, and by doing so we test our own Theory of Mind. Whereas real living people are extremely complicated and contradictory, our storied selves are necessarily less so (as Art is inevitably a reduction of real life with its vast and infinite interactions), enabling us to more easily grasp and essentially fine-tune our observations and calculations of others. Stories, and their interpretation, allow us to flex our Theory of Mind, and to improve our assessments and predictions.

As we will see, elements within the trickster stories reveal much of what has just been discussed: the struggle between the dispositional system (which causes behavior to occur in more automatic and primitive ways) and the mapmaking system (which is more "deliberative" and necessary for higher levels of "conscious" thought). Trickster often acts in a dispositional manner (on instinct) with little deliberation and consciousness. Yet his actions are always played out against other members of society who are highly conscious of social codes and taboos. Trickster's Theory of Mind is usually primitive, though he has to have *some* Theory of Mind to outwit his enemies, which happens frequently. Trickster can be a kind of transitional fossil showing us from whence we've come while not quite having arrived at where we are.

10

THE BRAIN OF GOD

The belief in God has often been advanced as not only the greatest, but the most complete of all the distinctions between man and the lower animals. It is however impossible, as we have seen, to maintain that this belief is innate or instinctive in man. On the other hand a belief in all-pervading spiritual agencies seems to be universal; and apparently follows from a considerable advance in the reasoning powers of man, and from a still greater advance in his faculties of imagination, curiosity and wonder.

—Charles Darwin, *The Descent of Man*

The creation of the mythic universe demanded the invention of two planes—the physical and the spiritual—a dualistic universe. The mythic world of stories would exist alongside the world of cuts and scrapes, broken bones, blood, weaponry, love, jealously, and hate, though elements of daily life bleed into the spiritual realm as well. The mythic world was something new, for it was "beyond," and could only be reached through dreams and visions, induced by sleep, trance, deprivation, hallucinogenic pharmacopeias, prayers, meditation, music, oratory, ritual, or songs.

The first physical evidence we have of the mythic mind coming into play is from the cave paintings, bone placements, burials, and carvings from around 40,000 to 50,000 years ago, but the fact that all of us stem from African ancestors some 150,000 years ago, and all share the same abilities in language, music, art, and mythology, shows that artistic/ mythic thought first developed with human beings in Africa before the great diaspora that led to our species populating the rest of the world. Most artifacts do not remain preserved; even fewer are ever found.

Dualistic thinking is a long-held notion in the Western world, but it is certainly not limited to it. Dualism is found in Judaism, Christianity, and Islam, and can be traced to the Persian dualism between Ormuzd and Ahriman,[1] (the good and evil powers that established Zoroasterism), as well as through Plato, and even the founders of science, such as Descartes—who believed in the mind/body split. But splitting everything into halves is common to the human mind, and dualism can be found around the world. Consequently, dualities surface everywhere: night and day; life and death; good and bad; man and woman; male and female; sun and moon; black and white; left and right; friend or foe; plant and animal; man and animal; man and nature; stop and go; happy and sad; young and old; guilty and innocent; nature and nurture; yin and yang, and on and on.

The most likely underlying reasons for carving the universe into binary units stem from two sources—the biological brain interacting with the environment to find the easiest methods of making value judgments, and the preference throughout the animal kingdom for symmetry. For our ancestors, there would have been little value in knowing that the universe consisted of eleven possible dimensions. Hominids on the African savannah had to make decisions instantly regarding survival, and this decision making was facilitated by emotion through the limbic system, which instigated action. A snake is about to strike you—run. Slicing the world into dual segments is a very efficient way for a brain to work fast. This is good; that is bad. A particular food could sustain you or make you sick. You were either the potential meal of another animal, or it was a potential meal for you. You could trust someone or you couldn't. A member of the opposite sex seemed like a good catch or someone to avoid.

Symmetry in nature is also an integral aspect of the biological world, with most animals being members of Bilateria, meaning they have a front and back as well as an upside and downside. The first creatures to exhibit this evolved some 550 to 600 million years ago. Symmetry is a marker for health. Biologists Thornhill and Moller found that those animals lacking symmetry had significant reductions in health and ability to have offspring.[2] Magnus Enquist and Anthony Arak found that "the existence of sensory biases for symmetry may have been exploited independently by Natural Selection acting on biological signals": in other words, the deep-seated preference for symmetry is both ancient and genetic.[3] There are two sides to every story, and our categorizing brains want to place things where they think they belong. Of course, the massive human brain with its neocortex is quite capable of seeing beyond such simple equations, but dualistic thought is still employed on a daily basis by all of us. It was Levi-Strauss and structuralism that first revealed this binary aspect of human thought, that (according to J. R. Rayfield) "the unconscious mind, has a certain structure that is manifested in all symbolic systems, i.e., all aspects of culture and even in the natural world."[4] Derrida, on the other hand, was preoccupied with "undermining the oppositional tendencies that have befallen much of the Western philosophical tradition . . . revealing the dualistic hierarchies they conceal."[5] Dualistic and hierarchical thought certainly can be oppressive, as the deconstructionists like Derrida claimed, but at the same time they are intrinsic. This does not mean that we are sentenced to see everything in simple oppositions; the freedom to rebel from such restriction is also part of what trickster tales reveal. The protean ability, an animal's potential to do the unexpected, which includes thinking the unexpected, is also part of our genetic makeup.

POTHEISM/MONOTHEISM AND THE SEARCH FOR MEANING

Religion is one of the true universals for humans. It is found in every culture on earth. In Zoroasterism, Christianity, Islam, and other religions associated with state-level societies, the dualities of good and evil are usually interpreted as sharply defined polarities, represented by opposing deities. But in most primal cultures the godhead, as well as the pantheon, is both good and evil at once, containing the essential elements of Trickster, who mitigates between the polar extremes. Actually, if we examine even the Old Testament more closely, we find that the Jewish god *too* embodies many negative traits as well (playing a trick on Mankind, kicking Adam and Eve out of the Garden; sending a flood; confusing the languages, and then we have references to "sons of god" going down and having sex with human females—and all of these betray trickster-like behavior). Trickster tales are an integral part of the mythic literature attempting to answer things like: Is the Creator good or evil? Does he behave for the good of Man, or is Man just a plaything the gods can destroy at their whim, without consequence? And where does morality fall into all of this? Socrates put it this way: "Is conduct right because the gods command it, or do the gods command it because it is right?" Are moral prescriptions relative or absolute?

Scientific methodology has allowed us to tease out the primal secrets that eluded us when trying to answer these questions through myth. Hence, we human beings have come a long way from the time when Jehovah could get angry with us for simply building a tower of mud reaching a few stories into the sky and confuse our tongues. Yet, even through we have gone to the stars and discovered the double helix of DNA, the quest for "God" goes on, though the definition for him or her has certainly changed. One would be hard-pressed to find very many top scientists who believe in an anthropomorphic Zeus or Yahweh, but even the search for unification in physics is part of the historic quest to uncover the ultimate forces that brought us here, which in tribal times meant deities.

The beginnings of science actually involved the search for God though his creations, as it was often men of the cloth who set out to find, through the particulars of nature, the hand of God in their design. Minute observation of phenomena was key to this search. The early religious men who developed what came to be science were radicals in that they dared to look for answers outside the pages of sacred texts, looking instead at the intricacies of nature itself. But they were surprised by what they found—like why did God make 10,000 species of beetle? Why did God make an untold number of parasites who seemed to have no other function than to devour us or make us miserable? Greater examination led to greater doubt. But it was not until Darwin that the real split between science and religion came to stay for good, for natural selection had no reason to keep God in the picture. But, as we can see today, religion has not withered away due to logic. Since the publication of *The Origin of Species*, many people have struggled to make coherent a worldview that takes into account the knowledge of science and the older worldviews based upon myth. Nearly every kind of argument has been invented so that evolutionary theory and religion can get along, such as *maybe God got the whole thing going,* or *possibly Adam and Eve were really hominids whom God gave souls,* as if there *must* be some way of reconciling myth and science. Then again, fundamentalists from every religion have dismissed science altogether, except when it comes to utilizing it to drive their cars, watch digital televisions, get medications, or fly somewhere else they want to be. Yet, for those who have the kind of minds in which truth cannot be so easily compartmentalized, the essential problems between science and religion have not gone away. For if the universe developed from natural causes that can be explained through the long and slow process of evolutionary change, who needs the hand of God? Educated people around the world, when confronted with the fact that the Jewish stories that make up the Old Testament were probably only written down some 2,600 years ago, in a world that is billions of years old, inevitably reach the conclusion that there is a disconnect between mythic explanations and scientific ones. But ironically, now that science has taken us to the point where we can begin to coax out the secrets of the brain itself, once again it is scientists who are leading the search for God. But they are not looking skyward. Rather, they have been looking into the synapses to try and discover how and why we came up with the notion in the first place. From the standpoint of *survival,* of natural selection, is there a reason for religion to exist?

WHY GOD?

For some twenty years, I had held in my head a theory that in many ways echoes that expressed in Matthew Alper's *The "God" Part of the Brain.* Alper's journey in search of God is in many ways my own. Having grown up in the Bible Belt culture, from the earliest moments I can remember I was immersed in the Bible-thumping old-time religion of my family and community. I loved the music, drama, and communal nature of that culture, and until I was a teenager I had a fairly absolute belief and imagined a life devoted to the Lord. The emotional part of this training is not easily put aside, and to this day there are few things I love more than singing the old hymns I learned as a child. Yet, around sixteen I began, like many teens, to question. The thesis I finally developed to explain religion went like this: Human beings, who having accidentally developed brains that were much too large for their own good (in that we think too much), suddenly had to face the prospect of their own demise. This was devastating knowledge, and from the fear of death religion sprang up in humans to give them peace. The mythic world was created by mankind in order to give hope and meaning to people living in a world they were now all too conscious of being temporary. They were aware of being aware, and they were aware that they would die. In order to survive, early humans needed some mechanism to counteract the knowledge of death, and this mechanism was religion.

Matthew Alper's scenario for how religion develops along these lines includes an added twist at the end: that god is a genetic trait from which developed a kind of organ in the brain—"A God Part of the Brain" that in culture after culture caused mankind to create the deities and religions that surround them.[6] Reading Alper's story gave me a sense of dejavu, for I certainly related to his progression toward a scientific explanation. But I no longer agree with his conclusion of how religious thought developed in our species—even though I had held a similar one for so long. While I agree that religion does many things that help avert fear, that religion often creates a sense of purpose, leads to feelings of cohesion and tranquility for the people and communities that practice it, I don't think that is how it started, just as I don't see that getting God into the genes is possible.

In order for that theory to work, there would have had to have been a time in the distant past where humans quite suddenly became acutely aware of their mortality (due to a relatively quick increase in brain size or cognitive ability). And with this knowledge they would have had to start despairing to the point where life itself no longer mattered. The non-god-believing hominids would have had to begun jumping off cliffs into the abyss to put an end to it all. At the same time, a few male believers who found "god" (through some change in their genetic code—which had not been found in the overall population) would suddenly have turned so suddenly charismatic in their life-affirming positive energy that they would have attracted the many females that flocked to them, thereby spreading these god genes wildly through the population. (Just like patriarchs of old—Abraham, with his harem—or King Solomon with his 700 wives). The believers would have won and instilled in their descendents the God gene.

I don't think so. Whatever the timeline of our mental rise to religious thought, it didn't happen overnight, and it hardly seems as though a specific gene for a belief in God could have developed and been so powerful to override the other physical and mental attractors that our species had developed for enticing sex. Plus, when it comes to sex, we are almost always talking about very young people in ancient times— and as we know now—until the age of twenty-five the brain is not fully developed. Risk assessment is notoriously skewed until then, as the brain has not developed the ability to reliably predict danger. This is one of the prime reasons the young make good soldiers: they will go into war thinking they're invincible to spears or arrows or guns. It's also why insurance rates are so staggering for youthful drivers: they get into more accidents because they do more stupid things than older people. They think they're going to live forever. The majority of those who would really need religion to give them peace of mind would be past the prime age for reproduction, and then it would be too late to get many of their genes into the pool anyway.

WHAT CAUSED RELIGION?

Just because religion mighty supply us with some benefits in relieving stress, it does not mean that such benefits are the cause of religion. In addition, not all religions give the assurance that Christianity or Hinduism does. (In Christianity, the ego and body remain intact as permanent fixtures in an everlasting life. In Hinduism, the end of karmic law is the final extinction of the self and a final end to suffering.) Some cultures offer a dim view of the afterlife. Life after death for the Lakota is ill defined. The soul goes up to the Milky Way. The "heaven" of the Nez Perce is hardly a "heaven" at all. Rather it is a shadowy world without joy, where people sit it semi-darkness. It's not always the case that religion offers a panacea to the ills of this world or a sense of peace to alleviate our fear of death. Nor do all religions offer paths of increasing wisdom, or courses of instruction that continue from one stage to the next—with the hope of attaining enlightenment, or at least contentment. Some religions strike fear into the hearts of their believers. In Christianity, this is certainly the reason we have Satan and hell. Even if believers can feel the certainty of an eternal reward, knowing that one's friends or loved ones who are not believers will burn forever in excruciating torture is not a very consoling thought. (The Gnostic *Gospel of St. Peter* actually has Christ telling the apostle this secret: that those in Hell will eventually get out).

In most tribal religions, the gods play little to no part in morality, judgment, reward or punishment. They exist, like other aspects of nature, without being sources of goodness or ethical revelation. They are put up with, or they are burdensome, requiring sacrifices to prevent the people from being pelted with volcanic rocks or left to starve because of drought, or drown in a flood. They are very "human" in their desires, lusts, and political machinations. They are not meant for universal consumption (every tribe has their own gods for themselves), and their concern is not for humanity but their particular group.

It's true that religions of every stripe involve music, singing, communal fellowship, group cohesion, stories that explain the meaning of the world with highly charged emotion. If you were a Quaker that emotion might lead to peace and tranquility. If you were living in the world of the Aztecs that emotion would probably be one of sheer terror, where the religious elite regularly cut out the living hearts of victims. For not all religions eliminate anxiety (the base of Alper's hypothesis). And while sometimes religion can bring out what we think of as the best in people—an altruistic spirit, concern for the poor and less fortunate, love for one's fellow Man, and tolerance—religion, as we all know, can also instigate brutality, war, torture, rape, genocide, conquest, annihilation, and the worst kinds of intolerance. Even Christianity, based on the teachings of a Jewish "rabbi" who preached *turn the other cheek* instead of an eye for an eye and a tooth for a tooth, has been used for hundreds of years to condone mistreatment, even genocide, against Jewish people. Religion is often the utmost specimen of contradiction in our species.

ORIGINS OF RELIGION

It could be that religion arose like the arts: those who developed incredible shamanistic powers became the most powerful people in the tribal hierarchy and consequently were able to attract a greater number of mates. But if the ethnological record from contemporary tribal peoples is any indication, this doesn't seem likely. Shaman, or medicine men, though given a good deal of respect in tribal cultures, and at times having opportunities for extra sexual favors due to their weird charisma, are on the other hand often seen as being a little crazed. They are often lost in their own visions, obsessed with their spiritual path, which is certainly not of this world, and there's not much in that repertoire that would make them prime candidates for husbands. They tend to be the most introspective members of the tribe—not the ones bringing home the bacon.

I believe it most likely that religion stemmed from the emotional and schema/categorizing properties of the brain itself, and specifically with our Theory of Mind. The limbic system of the brain, having to do with emotion, long ago in our ancient hominid ancestors likely led to the development of ritualistic communal celebrations, as we saw in the rain dances of chimpanzees, which coincided with the development of music. Our hominid ancestors reacted to the natural environment with awe, which is a kind of "spiritual" state. Music led to language, which played upon the pre-existing pattern of schema: basic cause and effect scenarios arising in the subconscious brain constructed for survival. Once parable/stories entered into true speech, the basic cause and effect patterning of the mind, when pointed to the larger questions (as a result of an expanded brain), intuitively began to make connections that had an undercurrent of dualistic logic.

In order to have a story, there has to be conflict. Conflict and personal agency are embedded in the structure of our sentences: *an actor acts.* We anthropomorphize. Our Theory of Mind is rampant. Origin myths are based upon the idea that willful intelligent agents cause things to happen. Humans were accustomed to seeing the world through the lens of personal intent. Your neighbor gets mad and throws a stone at you. Stones don't just come your way without someone wanting to inflict pain. When a rock comes tumbling at you down a mountain, *someone* must be doing that. When you're sick, there has to be a reason—an evil spirit was sent into you by your enemy. Likewise, natural disasters are caused by gods who are displeased. This is basic cause and effect. But this also brings up another problem connected to Theory of Mind: Confirmation Bias. Studies in neuroscience have shown repeatedly that the conclusions we believe are the ones that taint our sense of the world. We have bias. We stand where we sit. To change the worldview one was born with takes monstrous effort and self-control. Science itself is based on the belief that humans are capable of such self-regulation, through the requirement of verifiable information and peer review. But a dispassionate look at phenomena does not come naturally, and in the course of human life on earth science has only existed for a relative split second. Most of the time humans have been incapable of divesting themselves of their own limited perspectives and the mythic systems they were born into.

OTHER EXPLANATIONS

There are other explanations for religious thought, and these can further help to explain ways in which religion developed in our early ancestors. Even before stories of deities came into existence there were feelings that helped to drive a movement toward religious experience and cultural expression. Neural properties in the brain leading to shamanistic episodes, as well as the impact of dreams, visions, hallucinogenic drugs, and out-of-body experiences resulting from trauma or epilepsy could all have all played a part in affecting sensibilities that came to be thought of as occurrences operating from another plane. These forces are well documented in both religious and scientific literature and there is no doubt that they played an important role in establishing perceptions that helped to confirm early Man's belief in the duality of the physical and spiritual worlds. In order to cross over to the non-material dimension, everything from fasting and not drinking water (as in the Vision Quests of traditional Plains Indian tribes) to drugs such as peyote (used in the Native American Church) are and have been utilized to facilitate visionary states. While spending forty days and forty nights in the dessert would probably entice anyone to see visions (as did Jesus); forty days and nights on a boat full of two-of-every-kind of animal might indeed make one take up drink, (as did Noah after the flood). Cannabis has been used for religious purposes in the Middle East; Psilocybin mushrooms are used in Mesoamerica; the Amanita Muscaria mushroom is still used in shamanistic practices of Siberia, and the list could go on and on. Even coffee has a legendry connection with Catholic monks who, in ancient times, discovered that the drink allowed them to keep awake during prayers.

From the recent perspective of neuroscience, there have been many questions raised about the brain's role in seeing or creating god. The notion of the gene for God has been taken up by many more than Matthew Alper. Dean Hamer's *The God Gene*, published a few years before Alper's book, claims that religious thought is hardwired into our DNA to provide humans with "an innate sense of optimism" as they live with the awareness that death is "ultimately inevitable."[7] In 1997 Dr. Vilayanur Ramachandran delivered a paper, "The Neural Basis of Religious Experience," which said that the circuitry of the brain may have a good deal to do with religious thought: "If these preliminary results hold up, they may indicate that the neural substrate for religion and belief in God may partially involve circuitry in the temporal lobes, which is enhanced in some patients."[8] As Michael Shermer wrote in *The Humanist* regarding Ramachandran's discoveries,

> Using electrical monitors on subjects' skin (a skin conductance response commonly used to measure emotional arousal), Ramachandran and his colleagues tested three types of "emotional stimuli"—religious, violent, and sexual—in three populations: temporal lobe epilepsy (TLE) patients who had religious pre-occupations, normal "very religious" people, and normal non-religious people. In the latter two groups, Ramachandran found skin conductance response to be highest to sexual stimuli; in the first group the response was strongest to religious words and icons, significantly above the religious control group. Ramachandran considered three possible, but not mutually exclusive, hypotheses to explain his findings: that the mystical reveries led the patient to religious beliefs; that the facilitation of connections between emotion centers of the brain, like the amygdala, caused the patient to see deep cosmic significance in everything around him or her that is similar to religious experiences; that there may be neural wiring in the temporal lobes focused on something akin to religion. Other research tends not to support the first hypothesis, which leaves the latter two the likeliest explanations of the findings. Psychiatric and neurological patients who experience hallucinations, for example, do not necessarily exhibit religious propensities, but TLE patients, when shown religious words—as well as words with sexual or violent connotations—showed much higher emotional response to the religious words.[9]

Ramachandran's research gives scientific credence to claims long made by a number of theological commentators that a good many religious

saints, from Paul to Joan of Arc, were probably experiencing brain seizures when afflicted by acute religious visions.

Andrew Newberg, in *Why God Won't Go Away: Brain Science and
the Biology of Belief*, states his belief that an "evolutionary perspective
suggests the neurobiology of mystical experience arose, at least in part,
from the mechanism of the sexual response,"[10] and indeed, in ancient
times sexual practices were often associated with religious rituals.
Michael Persinger in *Neuropsychological Bases of God Beliefs*[11] has a
theory based on trauma which causes the brain to misinterpret information as mystical or out-of-body. He has developed a device which is
essentially a helmet equipped with electromagnets which produces a
field that causes micro seizures from overactive neutrons in the temporal lobe of the brain giving people religious sensations that range from
out-of-body experiences to experiencing angels or aliens. (Here it is
quite obvious the ways in which culture dictates what kind of religious
icons become available during a religious experience. A Lakota Indian in
ancient times, on the Great Plains of North America, would not see the
Virgin Mary, but rather the White Buffalo Calf Maiden.) Rick Strassman in *The Spirit Molecule* thinks that a single compound, DMT, found
in the pineal gland in the interior of the brain can account for religious
feeling.[12]

In all of these explanations, the brain is "tricked" somehow into interpreting senses that are skewed. These interpretations are visionary
and usually occur only to individuals, not groups, but the main notion
important to science is that the inner world of a person experiencing
religious conversion does not match with the exterior world of an observer watching them. While mass hallucinations have been reported
in history, they are infinitely rarer than the greater number of personal
perceptions of religious transformation caused by a variety of physical
and mental states—and some of them are known to have been initiated
through ingesting fungi or molds in food that had hallucinogenic properties. (A similar instance of the brain being tricked is what occurs in
cases of synaesthesia, where the brain sees colors that can be tasted and
sounds seen—a genetic occurrence—which has been touted as another
possible cause as an antecedent for religion.) Whatever the causes of
religious states, many have attested fiercely to their validity, just as many

others have attested to having seen ghosts, aliens, or other paranormal occurrences.

Whether religious mythology is seen and felt as verifiable truth or as metaphor, the stories stemming from the religious imagination have been the foundation of world literature. Religious literature has acted upon the minds of billions of people across the globe. Stepping back and looking at the trickster (Trickster almost always being a religious personage, a deity of some kind) tales from a global perspective, another aspect of these stories lies in their ability to shine a light on the mind from which religion sprang. Through a Cognitive Narrative critical approach to literature, stories can be examined from the perspective of evolutionary psychology and neuroscience in order to mine the brain for evidence of our ancient selves that is still a part of our psychology today. The trickster elements we see in gods around the world testify to the similar ways people have tried to confront the questions of our existence.

⑪

THE TRICKSTER OF MYTHOLOGY

We call literature one of the last frontiers because it is an easily documented fact: choose any subject relevant to humanity—philosophy, anthropology, psychology, economics, political science, law, even religion—and you will find a rapidly expanding interest in approaching the subject from an evolutionary perspective.

—Jonathon Gottschall and David Sloan Wilson

If others had not been foolish, we should be so.

—William Blake

The soap opera of human life, whether in the form of gossip or mythology, has been the stuff of oral literature since song and story were born. Nothing fascinates our species more than sex and love. The Trojan War began because of the beauty of Helen, and the first complete mythological story known—Gilgamesh (a trickster)—is infused with sexuality and love between men and men, and men and the gods. If mythic stories are reflections of our biological brains and our evolutionary past, we should see many of the aforementioned themes from the previous chapters being brought into play in the various trickster tales from unrelated cultures around the world. We should see something of the triune brain (the reptilian, the mammalian, the higher brain) that is contradictory at times; the workings of natural selection (fitness preferences, sex drive, promiscuity existing within pair-bonding) and sexual selection (the development of language and music as courtship behaviors); ethics (questions regarding the nature of ethical behavior, good, evil, and the nature of the gods). We should also see reflections in the stories of hierarchy and dominance in human interactions, since these are known to be wired into the brain. Since men and women evolved in tribal life with a clear split in work roles, we should as well see disparities in behavior between the roles of men and women: differing biological sexual roles and different roles in culture, which include themes of procreation, fidelity, paternity, familial obligations, and adherence to cultural taboos.

Trying to define Trickster in a tale where a "trickster" emerges is itself *tricky* in that there are no hard and fast boundaries in which the various aspects of Trickster can be completely defined or contained. As looked at previously, the notion of universal figures in literature have often been rebuked in the academy. Dario Sabbatucci says that the idea of a "trickster" is a "monstrous abstraction" that "puts the final lie to cross-cultural studies."[1] But as I began this argument, I stated my belief that there is a collection of traits, often bundled together, that are coherent enough for us to call "Trickster," a designation of a mythic and appropriated character that represents evolutionary forces upon a universal human brain/mind. In terms of just what these trickster traits may be, I want to begin with the "Historical Overview of Theoretical Issues: The Problem of the Trickster," wherein Doty and Hynes develop six overall traits that help to define the nature of Trickster, even though any particular manifestation of Trickster may contain only one or more:

1. the fundamentally ambiguous and anomalous personality of the trickster. Flowing from this are other features as
2. deceiver/trick-player
3. shape-shifter
4. situation-invertor
5. messenger/imitator of the gods
6. sacred/lewd bricoleur.[2]

(For an excellent delineation of various trickster types see Orrin Klapp's lists of heroes, villains, and fools in American culture in *Heroes, Villains, and Fools: The Changing American Character*; regarding women, see 199–200 of Marilyn Jurich's *Scheherazade's Sisters*.)

Looking at Doty and Hynes's list I would like to reiterate the fact that many trickster figures *are also* gods, or are one of a pantheon of gods (not just messengers of the gods), and that they have an essential and honored place in human cultures. It can also be, as in Greek mythology, that many of the gods have trickster attributes—from Zeus to Hermes— in that they exhibit one or more of the trickster traits, such as insatiable libido, creative power, and natures both devious and magnanimous. (To be clear, Trickster isn't always a deity; in some cultures, such as the Hopi, the Coyote trickster is seen as just a pest; though to the neighboring Navajo, Coyote is divine.)

In physical shape, the trickster of mythology often takes the form of an animal, such as Coyote, Rabbit, Spider, and Raven, in North America; Spider or Tortoise in Africa; while in China he is the Monkey King. There are numerous other incarnations of him that exist in oral literature worldwide. Then again, he is never completely animal, for he is really human—he is a *human animal*—and in the case of the Greek and Roman gods he often appears in different forms, shape-shifting, altering himself at will, utilizing a disguise, mask, or the body of any species of animal in order to deceive those around him. The various trickster figures of the many Bushman tribes, for example, can transform themselves into "human to animal and back, or from one animal species to another," and Trickster can change his social condition from story to story by in some cases having a "wife or wives, child or children, an extended family, and in some stories his family members (from the same tribe) are 'ancillary trickster figures' as well."[3] The various Bushman tricksters also typify the range of complex trickster personas "ranging from lewd prankster to divine creator; goblin to god; human to jackal; incarnation with the lowest animals, the louse, to Spirit Keeper of the highest, the eland [possessing] . . . contradictory and confounding traits."[4] The Viking trickster/god Loki, also with a number of wives and mistresses, can also change sex and shape at will. Thus, he can give birth as well as beget offspring. The eight-legged horse of Odin, Sleipnir, was born of Loki in the shape of a mare. In one story, Loki even eats the heart of an evil woman and grows pregnant. He fights with Heimdall in the shape of a seal for the possession of the Brísingamen necklace, and later, he sneaks into Freyja's residence in the form of a fly to steal the same precious object for Odin. According to an early poem, Odin and Loki had mixed their blood as foster brothers. "It has been suggested that Loki was a hypostasis of Odin, or at least that he represents Odin's darkest side. He seems to symbolize 'impulsive intelligence,' together with an irrepressible urge to act and an unpredictable maliciousness."[5]

In the Pacific Northwest, Raven shape-shifts so that he can be born to the god's daughter, in his quest to bring light to the people.[6] The "Tibetan trickster Agu Tompa, puts on the robes of a nun so that he can invade a cloister and make love with all the nuns."[7] The Winnebago trickster takes an elk's liver to make a vulva and elk kidneys to make breasts, changing himself into a woman so that so he can marry the chief's son, from whom he gets pregnant and has three kids before he is found out to be the male trickster.[8] The Greek trickster Hermes, a thief, transforms himself into mist to get through the key-hole of the door so he won't get caught.[9] Ananse, the West African trickster, "is free to modify his own bodily parts and those of others and to shift them around according to whim or need."[10] Orgo, another West African trickster, unites himself with his mother by entering her mouth and leaving again through her vagina.[11] In a Navajo tale, Coyote gets pulverized, cut to pieces, decimated time and time again, yet continually he comes back to life, which also happens in numerous Hopi Coyote stories. In a similar vein, in a Winnebago tale, Trickster burns his anus and eats his own intestines, but once again miraculously returns for more adventures. The Australian Aboriginal trickster, Rainbow Serpent, "undergoes endless transformations, from vastly pregnant cosmic giant, to a blind woman, to a man with daughters, to an ordinary looking snake."[12]

These are just a few of the shape-shifting behaviors of tricksters from around the world, for, as Doty and Hynes say, the

Trickster appears on the edge or just beyond existing borders, classifications, and categories . . . the trickster is cast as an "out" person, and his activities are often outlawish, outlandish, outrageous, out-of-bounds, and out-of-order. No borders are sacrosanct, be they religious, cultural, linguistic, epistemological, or metaphysical. Breaking down division lines, the trickster characteristically moves swiftly and impulsively back and forth across all borders with virtual impunity. Visitor everywhere, especially to those places that are off limits, the trickster seems to dwell in no single place but to be in continual transit through all realms marginal and liminal.[13]

Paul Radin, in his seminal book, *The Trickster,* one of the first and the most influential books on trickster studies, says

> Trickster is at one and the same time creator and destroyer, giver and negator, he who dupes others and who is always duped himself. He wills nothing consciously. At all times he is constrained to behave as he does from impulses over which he has no control. He knows neither good nor evil yet he is responsible for both. He possesses no values, moral or social, is at the mercy of his passions and appetites, yet through his actions all values come into being.[14]

The trickster can be both the initiator of pain or the merciful healer who takes pain away. He can, through his actions, become a savior, alleviating the sufferings of the world and as Jung says, "transform the meaningless into the meaningful" while still being a deviant. Indeed in Jung's essay "On the Psychology of the Trickster Figure" he states how alike the shaman (or medicine-man-woman/healer) is to the trickster figure:

> There is something of the trickster in the character of the shaman and medicine man, for he, too, often plays malicious jokes on the people, only to fall victim in his turn to the vengeance of those whom he has injured. For this reason his profession sometimes puts him in peril of his life. Besides that, the shamanistic techniques in themselves often cause the medicine man a good deal of discomfort, if not actual pain. At all events the "making of a medicine-man" involves, in many parts of the world, so much agony of body and soul that permanent psychic injuries may result. His "approximation to the saviour" is an obvious consequence of this, in confirmation of the mythological truth that the wounded wounder is the agent of healing, and that the sufferer takes away suffering.[15]

Whether it be taking on the sins of the world through a sacrificial scapegoat, as in the case of Jesus on the cross, or the dancers in a Plains Indian Sun Dance, or sacrificing through some private personal act of deprivation, such as fasting, meditation, or prayer, humans have universally seen such actions as important ways by which mental and physical illness can be tricked away from the people and the world purified from its woes. Though it is also true that these actions are undertaken to make right what the trickster Gods have wreaked upon humanity in the first place. Trickster techniques are used for dealing with Trickster gods.

That the religious virtuoso who undergoes such trials and tribulations is actually another manifestation of the trickster can be both noticed or unnoticed in the various societies in which these rituals exist, but the shaman or healer intentionally deceives the demons by driving them out (as Christ does in sending them into the swine before driving them over the edge of a cliff). The shaman fools the spirits who have no particular concern regarding the pains of men and women—who at times neither bring rain to the crops when it is needed, or bring so much rain that everything floats away in a flood.

So Trickster, while often a powerful deity, can also be an agent of revolution against the even more powerful gods, as Tricksters are notorious for shattering false idols, castigating the pompous, and castigating hubris.

WHY TRICKSTER?

We are dealing with an enigma when we try to analyze Trickster, for he is never easy to pin down as one persona or thing. He is more like Heisenberg's Uncertainty Principle—there is no certainty when you expect to find it. All you can say is that there is a probability of something occurring. And when you do find "it," it is in the form of energy; and energy, more than anything describes the trickster's power and flux.

The question of just why Trickster came to be, and why is he so prominent in world literature, has been addressed by a number of scholars before. Schoolcraft (1793–1864), who made a study of American Indian culture found "two gods in Indian theology which strongly [reminded him] of the old Persian dualism between Ormuzd and Ahriman, representatives of the good and evil powers in existence."[16] Making correlations between discovered native oral literature and Western literature (a search for universals) was common for scholars of that period, yet such ideas were almost always wrong. For the paradigms regarding how similar stories from around the world might be linked were flawed—the premise that they were caused by actual contact or were derivatives of older cultures. In the same way, many early scholars interpreted native forms as mimicking Western culture—such as the pyramids of Middle and South American stemming from Egypt, or the mounds and earth carvings of the Missippian Indian cultures being evidence of the lost tribe of Israel. It was assumed that neither architectural nor literary "marvels" could have been created by "primitive" Indians. Therefore, many early Europeans saw North American tricksters as incarnations of Satan. But the range of connotations of a character, such as Satan, from one tradition cannot be laid upon another without creating an incorrigible mess. (This is one reason many still find any search for universals annoying.) Coyote in any specific culture in North America would not carry the connotations (or baggage) of Satan in the Western tradition: fallen angel, pure evil, adversary to God, and so forth. (Indeed, as we have seen, Coyote often is a god himself who creates.) Distinctions must be made regarding the scope and limitations of cross-cultural analysis. In addition, it's often the case that even within particular cultures, mythic characters can be interpreted in quite different ways by different individuals. Cultures without writing are often quite happy to also have multiple versions of stories. Yet, even though localized stories and connotations exist, the fact remains that human minds around the world have come up with very similar mythological tales and mythological characters, which points to something universal in the human mind.

The father of American anthropology, Boas, steered clear of any sacred interpretation of Trickster by saying that Trickster "helps man only incidentally by advancing his own interests."[17] In Boas's interpretation, Trickster didn't have to have any noble qualities to do good, which was a convenient way to avoid controversy regarding the god/trickster nature of many deities, including Jehovah. The religious aspect of Trickster was just eliminated by Boas (Boas also put the Devil under the category of folkloric rather than religious).[18] On the other hand, in Europe Kurt Breysig brought Trickster squarely into the religious fold, as the link between the animistic belief system of earliest man (where animals were gods) to the anthropomorphic concept of god (that god is human-like). This was just the opposite of Brinton, who "interpreted the lecherous trickster as a later and corrupt version of an originally divine being."[19]

Paul Radin saw evolution in the trickster persona. He looked at the Winnebago stories as a cycle in which Trickster would, through his journey, eventually become the cultural hero—a savior hero who transformed over the course of a mythic cycle into a creature who would gain control of his desires and elemental cravings, transforming from rascal to messiah. This later culture hero has Christian overtones of the savior, which Jung brings up in his essay (contained in Radin's book), as we see the jealous and angry Jehovah, God of the Old Testament, who declares "an-eye-for-an-eye, a-tooth-for-a-tooth" give way to the "turn-the-other-cheek" Jesus of the New Testament. But Radin's idea of Trickster who evolves from an earlier, naughtier form of the godhead into something enlightened is an idea most scholars today do not take seriously—though this is not to say that in specific instances (such as the Judeo-Christian Jesus or the Chinese Monkey King) one might not find such an interpretation of a deity's altering character over time. The evolution Radin spoke of was based on misbegotten premises of an earlier age that saw history as a continual progression from primitivism toward civilization. The other fallacy with the evolving trickster thesis is that in it the essential element of Trickster is being lost, the fact that he is sacred and profane *at once*—not that he is moving from one state to another. Trickster is more akin to the concept of yin and yang—nonlinear and constantly contained within its other self.

Radin also gave a reason for the existence of trickster stories: they release stress. In support of this theory, it is true that many Native American cultures do have an edict stating that trickster tales can only be told in the winter. In previous times, winter was the period in which people in the frozen northern latitudes were forced to huddle together in wigwams, longhouses, or teepees, during cold dark months. Radin sees Trickster as a relief valve that can blow off the steam of social friction, when not even avoidance procedures could be guaranteed to solve social problems. By breaking societal taboos that everyone else must abide by, Trickster, through proxy releases through laughter the tensions of social proximity. This seems one credible aspect of Trickster's raison d'être. But anthropologist Levi-Strauss saw Trickster as another kind of relief valve, one that embodies "all complementary opposites, but in particular of that between immediate sexual gratification and the demands of civilization"[20] There may be some truth in this analysis as well, if one leaves out "civilization." For people in tribal societies are also faced with sexual proscriptions, for no tribal society on earth enjoys unbridled sexual freedom (even the few that have at certain times allowed for unrestricted sexual access outside of marriage bonds), for all have clear rules regarding sexual activity and marriage.

Victor Turner sees Trickster as a character at the margin: "liminal Trickster, the court jester, and the clown are related . . . in that they possess marginal status and bring into the social institution new possibilities,"[21] which is, I do believe, an important aspect of Trickster, one that I often refer to as Trickster's representation of a creative protean way of behaving—the ability to move without prediction. The only way to get away from Bre'r Fox is to do something unexpected—like asking him to throw you into a briar patch—out-of-the-box thinking. Another important factor regarding creativity that the Trickster represents is Neophilia, what Darwin thought as central to courtship displays, saying in *The Descent of Man*, "It would appear that mere novelty, or change for the sake of change, has sometimes acted like a charm on female birds, in the same manner as changes of fashion with us."[22] Trickster's constant shape-shifting is evidence of this—a constant turnover—constant novelty, creating interest, including sexual interest. The Trickster is a perpetual incarnation of change and surprise, doing the last thing expected, the most unpredictable action, coming like a thief in the night, violating the usual rules of going in through the door at a reasonable hour and first giving a knock. He zigzags when he runs, and by doing the improbable, elicits erotic attention and still usually escapes from his enemies.

Other interpretations include Robert Pelton's, that Trickster shows humans "individually and communally seizing the fragments of his experience and discovering in them an order sacred by its very wholeness"[23] (which may be true in some instances of tricksterism but certainly not in all), while Mary Douglass views Trickster as "dispelling the belief that any given social order is absolute and objective,"[24] an idea central to Post-Modernism and Deconstruction. I think this is true in that by taking us on a journey to the extremes, Trickster does call into question all rules and regulations—poking fun at the premise that the great energy of nature can be truly controlled.

Black Elk, the Sioux Holy Man, thought that the Heyoka trickster, through his humorous antics, could turn the people away from pain and danger, bringing laughter as medicine that could work even in the worst of circumstances to aid survival. Forgetting cold, hunger, pain, may just give one an edge toward making it to the next day, or the next, or the next, wherein relief might come. Humor itself may have been an important ingredient for survival for our early ancestors, something that helped them to face the frightening prospects of a future, where even if you did everything right and were lucky, you ended up dead. And lest we forget—Trickster is funny. This is a relief from stress that goes much further than Radin's summation, for here the stress is both physical and mental—everything from hunger to ennui. If Trickster wasn't funny, he would never have been so popular. What makes Trickster funny is that he is being pulled at from opposite psychological ends, which make him desire this as well as that—to have his cake and eat it too—being an insider and an outsider at the same time—not recognizing where boundary markers occur. The very fact of his having desires also makes him *tragically* funny, for as all humans know, our grasp is always impeded by our reach. Living with the knowledge of our ultimate limitation—death—humor allows us a temporary reprieve—a way of confronting the absurd without being defeated by our knowledge. For a moment, we as well as Trickster cope—surviving for the time being—with as much panache as possible.

The teaching of moral lessons has been another explanation from theorists for the existence of trickster stories, as the children who hear them learn in reverse—*not to do* what the trickster does—for in many stories (like the Hopi) Trickster comes to no good in the end because he has broken the societal taboos, though the pieces miraculously get put back together again for another telling. In other tales, such as the Northwest Coast story "We-gyet and his Wife," we see Trickster violating the sacred rules and getting his comeuppances, or in "Coyote and the Shadow People," where his impatience brings the permanence of death into the world. But in many of the stories the "moral" is much less clear or nonexistent. Rather, we are left with moral ambiguity—or the sense that Trickster exposes the fact that our brains are modular and contradictory. Some tales may be cautionary, many deal with moral issues, but it is rare to find them becoming mere "morality tales," as in Grimm's. Good and bad are usually a mixed and intertwined bag, with humor part of the mix. Hearing trickster stories is like listening to the basal ganglia (or the primitive brainstem) talking to the neocortex, as Trickster reveals our base motivations and desires. Trickster, in some cultures, also has a childlike innocence—not really Machiavellian intent—for complete consciousness has yet to occur—as in the brain of the fish or reptile—full of appetite, yet not calculating: often lacking in self-awareness altogether and engaging *because Trickster does not plan* his escapades, having no preconceived idea except to go forth. Our sympathies are most usually with him—as we admire his perseverance and continual optimism, his air of innocence and naiveté, which gives him great charm.

But there can be a dark side to Trickster, one that Jung calls the Shadow. In Freud's analysis, mental aberrations were thought to result from repression, and Jung's interpretation of the Shadow is akin to this. The Shadow exists behind a mask that says *that everything is fine*; but in not recognizing the Shadow (inside oneself) all hell can break loose. The theory of mental aberrations resulting from repressed sexual obsession, or other areas of restraint, are no longer taken seriously by Psychology, which has moved from armchair speculation into evolutionary-based science. But I think there is an element of truth here that I would reframe from the perspective of cognitive science and evolutionary theory. By telling the trickster stories we make fun of our own dominance struggles and our own brain wiring that goes from the neocortex to the amygdala to the basal ganglia and back again. By exposing the shadow, we are releasing the most primal impulses and fears that parts of the brain create, so that we might not do as the character in the famous Zen story does: falsely reach for the moon by trying to touch its reflection in the pond.

TRICKSTER BIOLOGICAL ORIGINS

In the broad sense, I think the trickster tales primarily reflect conflicts in the human brain that are a result of the evolutionary process: these stories reflect our biological selves. As far as having pre-wired contradictions we are not unique, but evolution of the neocortex and the parallel evolution of culture have given us much more to deal with than any other animal. Coming from the need for social communication, we, like our primate cousins, developed a large repertoire of signals to translate everything from mood to desire. Through rhythm, which became synchronized for group activity, music was born, which was amplified and selected for by the process of sexual selection. Music and language as song (music and words together) is an important tool for courtship as is language itself. At the same time, our hominid ancestors who had previously transferred from trees to savannah-living creatures, were developing larger and larger brains which necessitated entering into pair-bond mating practices, which led to the biological process of love— itself a kind of trick for the purpose of reproduction and the caring of the helpless young. As our ancestors began to communicate in greater ways, through an expansion of mirror cells, stories and characters came to be—including Trickster—who has never left us. For he represents all the struggles within our brains. When the Winnebago trickster's left hand fights with his right, we see a reflection of the old brain stem of desire conflicting with the neocortex (and societies' proscribed social codes). Trickster's constant search for sexual consummation reveals the male's outlandish biological self—millions of sperm available to impregnate multiple females—set against the female's one egg that she wants to protect. The male trickster sometimes succeeds in his promiscuity, but he often fails, and his failure unleashes a great deal of humor, for it points to that other evolutionary fact of our species—that pair-bonding is the most successful and responsible strategy for raising our young (responsibility is the thing Trickster rebels against the most). For as much as we want order we also desire liberation from it. When Trickster tries to make himself look better than he is, through changing shape to entice a female, we see the Handicap principle being played out, wherein it is up to the female to be able to detect a fraud. When we see Trickster playing music, singing, or wooing with words, we are seeing Courtship behavior in action, which probably initiated all the arts and may have developed our Ornamental Mind.

(12)

A SWATH OF TRICKSTER
STORIES FROM ORAL LITERATURE

No matter how much cats fight, there always seem to be plenty of kittens.

—Abraham Lincoln

SEX, DESIRE, AND THE BODY

Procreation is the driving force in evolution and the end to which our "selfish genes" are dedicated. Sex and love are the primary topics of literature, poetry, and song, and it should be no surprise that the trickster stories are the same. But what is surprising to Westerners when reading trickster stories from other cultures is the often loose and graphic nature of the tales, where the trickster's penis is neither hidden from view nor in any way tamed. The following stories from pre-literate cultures around the world attest to the trickster's sexual proclivity, his insatiable desire for every hedonistic activity, and his obsession with every bodily function. Considering the fact that Trickster's mental state is lust, the fact that he is usually male should not come as a shock. This is not always the case, and I will explore female trickster figures in the next chapter, but it is typical. The male's repertoire for courtship arts (like having a silver tongue with which to woo) stems from his subconscious desires to spread his seed and multiply his genes. But rather than merely condoning Trickster's masculine virility and wiliness, the trickster stories usually end up also mocking the male Trickster's persona as well, in one sense painting the rapscallion for what he is—often a low-down, good for nothing cheat. By exposing his male attributes, the trickster tales often include a hidden feminine critique of the male while also celebrating Trickster's phallic prowess—a contradiction of meaning and intent.

White missionaries often recoiled at the graphic nature of trickster tales when they first heard them, seeming to have no awareness of trickster stories from their own cultural traditions. This reaction caused real anxiety among tribal people who when asked to relate trickster tales to anthropologists told the stories with trepidation, fearing they'd be judged as "savages." Though nowadays the trickster in North America is a celebrated figure (especially in the form of Coyote, though almost always cleaned up; even a version of him was made into a well-known Warner Brothers cartoon: Wile E. Coyote). One can spot numerous images of Coyote all over the Southwestern United States—in gift shops taking the form of carvings, sculptures, ashtrays, refrigerator magnets, and as characters portrayed in stories and books written by both native and non-native writers alike. So, on the surface, he is "in." But my own experience while visiting American Indian territory is that there is still some hesitation in relating trickster stories to non-tribal members, primarily because of those old fears of being called "primitive." Of course, these connotations were instilled in Indian people through years of missionary work, but I think there is something else at work here as well. For the prudery we maintain in our culture is reflected to one degree or another in every culture on earth (I am not talking about Puritanical fanaticism). The reason Trickster is so popular in all of these cultures is because he openly *breaks* the sexual taboos that exist to impede sexual freedom. It's the shock value that makes people laugh (and remember that in many American Indian cultures, Trickster stories can only to be told in winter). If there were no proscriptions regarding sexual behavior, if they did not touch on dangerous territory, Trickster stories would be neither funny nor interesting. As Franchot Ballinger states,

In early times among the Klamath, obscene anal and erotic details were essential features of some myths (both Trickster and non-Trickster) and were recounted even in the presence of children. Native American playwright Hanay Geiogamah acknowledges that "among the boys" Trickster stories were commonly pornographic (Lincoln 75–76). Nevertheless, while these stories may have provided juicy entertainment, the social dangers and disorder attending or threatened by men's unbridled sexuality is at the heart of a number of Trickster tales.

Trickster's prodigious sexual appetites and energy are hilariously and powerfully dramatized by the gamut of their lusts and the size of their penises. The Yurok trickster, Wohpekumeu, to cite one instance, is so sexually robust and so promiscuous that he impregnates women with a mere glance. Because of his sexual threat, the people once literally leave him in the world alone, making him temporarily one of the few truly outcast tricksters.

No woman is safe for long from a Trickster's penis; not virgins or other men's wives, not his daughters, not his mother-in-law, not even his grandmother. Nor, consequently, is any social relationship or institution safe. Community well-being and harmony, friendship, marriage, family: all fall before Trickster's incorrigible penis. Sometimes a Trickster's sexual rapaciousness drives him to violate very specific tribal moral customs. . . . Human females are not his only victims; a buffalo cow mired in a wallow is on occasion as acceptable to a Trickster as a human woman. In a sense, he even sexually abuses men when in some stories he marries a chief's son. Thanks to his prodigious penis, Trickster even 'abuses' himself when he commits self-fellatio. The issue in many of these stories is not sexual victimization as such but rather the cruelty, self-deception, and absurdity of a man whose unrestrained sexuality poses a threat to the community. Such stories dramatize the power of human sexuality to whirl us beyond the boundaries of human social constraints.[1]

I think this is both true and not true at the same time. For Trickster is nothing but a whirl of opposites. Embedded in the Trickster tales is a world of sexual mindsets, fears, and taboos, many of which the tales confront either overtly or covertly. But it would be wrong to either reduce the stories to cautionary tales *or* to interpret them as condoning the behavior they depict. They are both simultaneously—on one hand celebrating the phallic while equally mocking that little hanging piece of flesh with a mind of its own. Of course, at the very heart of human folly lies sex, which is life, which drives us toward love and madness, dominance and status: a perfect place for humor to level our pretensions. Tribal people realized that we are like any other animals in physical mating, yet in all other aspects of sex (love, emotion, cultural taboos, responsibility) we act in opposition to "mere" animal lust. The Trickster stories reveal the tensions that the evolution of consciousness, conscience, and societal codes caused. The old reptilian brain, the mammal brain, and the new brain had to get along, even though they were often in a warring state. Creating stories and sharing them was a way of bringing out in the open those subconscious desires, making fun of them, and lessening their power to drive us mad, through laughter. What follows are Trickster stories that focus upon desire.

A note here must be made of how stories are related. Trickster stories throughout the Americas have been swapped, stolen, borrowed, or reworked, for we see some of the same plots being repeated in exact form or with derivations (such as Trickster and the ducks story). North American origin genres include Diver stories of creation, in which case a creature, such as Beaver, dives to the bottom of a lake and pulls up mud to make the first land. Another example would be Emergence tales, from the ancestors who originate from a hole in the earth, from another world—and in North America it is the fourth world into which they have arrived (as the primal number in American Indian cultures is four). Looking at the lineage of any particular mythic story gets even more complex when the dimension of borrowing between native and colonized cultures is added into the mix. Oftentimes, mythologies merge with one another, as we see throughout the Americas in regards to native and Christian influences. Elements of Christian mythology will often also creep into the translated accounts of native mythology, which in most cases were collected by European Christians. Sometimes this is due to the interpreters adding their own biases and commentary, and sometimes it is because native peoples have taken Christian stories and woven them into their own. Yet, even when such syncretism occurs, native mythic elements can often be discerned from the European by looking through the mask of the more recent Christian importation. A good case in point comes from a story by anthropologist Ruth Benedict, who, visiting the Zuni tribe of the Southwest United States in the 30s during a Christmas celebration, was surprised to find that when she followed the Indian people into the Catholic mission church, she was shocked to find at the alter, wooden statues of Joseph and Mary in a copulating position, which merged into the Christian mythology their original native elements of sexual energy and rebirth at the time of the winter solstice celebration.

But there are far too many creation and trickster stories worldwide for the process of borrowing to account for them all. In general, when very specific elements are the same in a story (as in the flood accounts of Gilgamesh and Genesis), we can be sure of direct borrowing—this being even more certain if there is a geographical or historical relationship. However, when stories are found in different parts of the world from cultures in which direct or indirect contact did not occur, the likelihood of borrowing approaches zero. One thing that makes Trickster tales so interesting is that we do see the same kinds of similar themes emerging in every culture on earth in these stories, regardless of individual and specific details—pointing to the fact that these types of stories are being generated again and again by the human mind, and that they are continually found to be a source of significance and enjoyment.

SOME TRICKSTER STORIES FROM AROUND THE WORLD

Coyote Marries a Man (Plains Cree, North America)

Coyote traveled to a new tribe where there was food and lots of people. A handsome man lived there named Not Enough Horses, who desired marriage, but none of the women there were good enough for him.

Coyote shape-shifted into a gorgeous woman to make this man marry him. Not Enough Horses fell for the female version of Coyote, they married, and Coyote bore three children, but no one was allowed to see them, until one day Coyote accidentally left them behind, and Not Enough Horses' mother discovered the children were wolf pups, not humans, and she began laughing, knowing that Coyote had played a trick and gotten his comeuppance for being so arrogant. Not Enough Horses left the village, determined to marry the first ugly woman that he saw, and he did. But once again, it was Coyote in disguise. He had married Coyote twice.[2]

This story deals with the ways in which the brain tricks itself to believe what it wants. As Robert Burton says in *On Being Certain*, belief in something has little to do with its validity: "Once firmly established, a neural network that links a thought and the feeling of correctness is not easily undone. An idea known to be wrong, continues to feel correct."[2] Bias becomes us, both through biology and culture, and this tale relates the problem of being myopic, while also dealing with the humor of lust and the importance of social standing.

Coyote and Beaver Exchange Wives (Cochiti, North America)

At Amatsushe they were living; Old Coyote and Old Coyote Woman lived on one side of the hill and Old Beaver and Old Beaver Woman lived on the other. They visited each other every night. One night it was snowing, deep, and Old Coyote said to his wife, "I shall go to Old Brother Beaver to invite him to go hunting, and to make plans for exchanging our wives."

When Coyote got there, he called, "Hello." Beaver answered, "Hello, come in and sit down." They sat together by the fireplace to smoke.

Coyote said, "I came to tell you we are to go hunting. If we kill any rabbits we'll bring them to our wives. I'll bring mine to your wife, and you can bring yours to mine."

"All right," Old Beaver agreed.

"You go first," said Coyote. "No, you go first. This is your invitation; you invited me," Beaver insisted.

"All right, I shall go early in the morning."

Coyote said to Old Beaver Woman, "In the morning I am going hunting for you."

"All right. I shall sing the song so that you will kill many rabbits."

Old Beaver Woman started to fix the supper. She wanted it ready for his return. Old Coyote was gone for the whole day. It was evening, and he did not come home at all. Sitting near the fireplace, Old Beaver Woman waited and waited. She started to sing her song: Old Coyote, Old Coyote, come sleep with me, Come have intercourse with me.

Old Beaver said, "What are you singing about? He won't kill anything, for he isn't any hunter." Coyote killed nothing, and Beaver Woman waited and waited but Coyote never came.

Next day it was Old Beaver's turn to go hunting. He went to tell Old Coyote Woman that she must wait for him, for he was going to hunt rabbits for her. "All right," she said. And he killed so many that he could hardly carry them.

In the morning Beaver came into Coyote's house and said, "Old Coyote Woman, here are the rabbits." She took them and said, "Thank you, thank you, Old Man Beaver."

They went straight into the inner room, and Old Man Coyote was left by himself in the front room. He was very angry. They gave him his supper, and when he had finished, they went in to bed.

Old Beaver Man started to have intercourse with Old Coyote Woman.

Old Coyote Woman cried out, and Old Coyote called out, "Old Beaver, don't hurt my wife." Old Coyote Woman answered, "Shut up, Old Man Coyote! It's because I like it that I'm crying out."

When he had finished, Old Beaver Man came out. He said to Old Coyote, "We won't keep bad feelings against each other; this was your plan. I shall always wait for you at my house whenever you want to visit me." And they were as good neighbors as ever.[3]

Embedded in this story is the difficult nature of the pair-bond, which is imperfect, as even the marriage ceremony and societal obligation are not enough to keep the wayward male from straying. As we have seen, there are very definite biological reasons for the pair-bond having developed and for keeping it intact over a long period of time: children. But a couple does not need to have children for all the emotions of marriage to be intact; those are given us at birth. Here, the male's desire to "control" access to his mate does not affect his desire for sexual novelty. The female's investment in the relationship, from an evolutionary standpoint, equals resources for her family which she will fight for. But here she outsmarts her lustful husband in her own trickster fashion, tricking the trickster, keeping him in his place so that he will not be thinking of another woman, so *he* will be jealous. On top of it, she gets the benefit of another man's ability to bring home the bacon.

The Winkte Way (Omaha, North America)

Winkte is the Sioux world for hermaphrodite or transvestite. Such people were also known as Berdaches in Indian literature. Iktinike and Rabbit are always chasing women, but sometimes, just for a change, they turn themselves into winktes, doing it the winkte way.

Iktinike and Rabbit were ambling about. By chance they met. "Hau, uncle," said Rabbit, "I was just thinking about you—and here you are!"

"Yes nephew, I am glad to see you," said Iktinike. "I have been thinking about you. Come along. Let's go someplace where nobody can see us."

"Why, uncle?"

"You are asking too many questions. Come along."

They went into the woods. "Friend," said Iktinike, "bend over. Let me get on top of you. Let's do it the winkte way."

"No, uncle," objected Rabbit. "You bend over and I get on top of you."

"No, young friend. I am the older. I go first. Respect your elders."

"On the contrary, "Rabbit insisted, "youth must be served. It is the younger who always go first."

They argued for a while. At last Iktinike lost patience. "All right, get on top of me." Rabbit did. "Oh, it hurts!" cried Iktinike. "Your che is very big!"

"No it isn't," said Rabbit. "Your onze is too tight." After only a few seconds, Rabbit got off Iktinike's back and ran off. Rabbit is very quick at that kind of thing.

As Rabbit was running off, Iktinike called after him: "Hey, come back! It's my turn now!" But Rabbit just continued running, laughing loudly. "That rotten, evil-smelling, bug-eyed fellow has played me false," Iktinike complained. "It's just like him. He always plays tricks on me and I fall for them."

Iktinike was furious. He would have liked to punish Rabbit, but Rabbit was too fast. He could not be caught. So all Iktinike could do was call Rabbit some very bad names. So Iktinike was walking toward home. He came to a place where some boys were playing stickball. Iktinike called out to them: "Hokshila," "what's new?"

"Nothing much, uncle," one boy answered. "Only that Rabbit came by here, telling everybody that he mounted you."

"Oh, he shamed me," thought Iktinike. "He's bad-mouthing me already!"

Iktinike went on. He came to a place where boys were gambling with plum pits. "Young brothers," Iktinike inquired, "what's new?"

"Nothing much. Rabbit came through here and told everybody how he got on top of you."

"Oh, no! That no-good, lying long-eared hlete is only spreading false rumors!"

Iktinike went on. He came to a place where boys were shooting with toy bows and arrows. "Hey, you kids, what's new?" *Iktinike wanted to know.*

"Only that Rabbit came through here, telling everybody that he used you in the winkte way."

"Ph, that split-nosed, stinking liar!" *cried Iktinike.* "Don't believe him!"

Iktinike hurried on. Suddenly he had to relieve himself. He squatted down, but instead of chesli, little baby rabbits popped out of his onze. "Oh, now! This is really too much! Cried Iktinike. "What next?"

Finally, he arrived at his home. His wife greeted him lovingly. She was in an amorous mood. "Let's tawiton," *she said.*

"Not tonight," *Iktinike declined.* "I've got a headache."[4]

Here we see Coyote doing what many tricksters around the world do, shape-shift between male and female forms, partially to allow for more varied sexual adventures. Coyote and Rabbit turn themselves into hermaphrodites or transvestites in order to have anal intercourse. But only Rabbit does the mounting in this case, and Coyote gets all the pain and none of the pleasure, so much so that he even has to turn down having sex with his wife. Part of what this story reveals is how sexual novelty is highly desirable for males of various species. From an evolutionary point of view, having the male be "over-sexed" is beneficial to any particular male's genes; that this urge spills over into homosexual activity on occasion makes little difference so long as most of the male's energies go toward procreation. For those who are born *winktes*, however, there is no evolutionary advantage; but nature is never perfect, and a wide variety of maleness and femaleness occurs naturally in animal and human populations. In addition, males of various species (even gorillas) will become homosexual temporarily if no females are present. Neuroscientist V. S. Ramachandran relates the following story in his book *The Tell-Tale Brain* about a psychological experiment known as the "Coolidge effect," named after President Calvin Coolidge. A sex-starved rat is put in a cage with a female and proceeds to copulate with her numerous times until he is so exhausted he can no longer move—that is, until another female rat is introduced, and then the male has sex with the new female all over again with the same zest as the first, until he is utterly exhausted and falls over. Put in yet *another* female rat and the male mates with her just as vigorously as he did the first and second. The Coolidge part of the story stems from a time when the president and first lady were visiting a chicken coop in Oklahoma. The first lady was shown around the grounds while the president was making a speech, and she was quite impressed to learn that the rooster serviced the dozens of hens every night, all night long. She then asked her guide to relate the same story about the rooster to the president once his speech making was over. The guide went with Mrs. Coolidge over to the president once his speech was over and told the president all about the rooster doing it all night and every night with the hens. The president asked, "With the same hen or different hens?" "Different hens," the guide promptly told him.

Legba (Fon, West Africa)

Legba denied that he had had relations with a mother and a daughter, but his parent [Mawu-Lisa] ordered him to undress. As he stood naked, Mawu saw how is penis was erect and said, "You have lied to me, as you have deceived your sister [Gbadu]. And since you have done this, I ordain that your penis shall always be erect, and that you may never be appeased." To show his indifference to his punishment, Legba began at once to play with Gbadu before their parent, and when reproached, merely pointed out that since his organ was always to remain erect, Mawu had herself decreed such conduct for him. That is why Legba dances, he tries to take any woman who is at hand.[5]

The erect male member is often a thing of humor and derision in many trickster stories. In this tale Trickster breaks cultural taboos about with whom one may have sex, and his punishment is a permanent erection. As mentioned previously, human males are one of the few mammals that do not have a penis bone, so there is no automatic erection without some mental arousal. The penis is a kind of red flag, revealing the mind of the man, but here that is taken away and the penis itself becomes as if it had a penis bone, never having a chance to go flaccid. Ironically, this only shows the true nature of Trickster who might as well have a penis bone or an erection all the time, as he is constantly ready for intercourse. This tale shows men to be who they are and the nature of their trickery neverending, as Trickster once again tries breaking sexual taboos by attempting sexual relations with his sister.

Coyote Visits the Women (Assiniboine, North America)

Coyote was wandering and came across a big lake with a village. When he got to the village he discovered that there were no men. When he asked about this, a woman told him.

"We don't know what you are talking about."

Inside the main lodge, he was told that a fox and a rabbit were "children," and they were wrapped onto a papoose board.

Coyote got a hard-on, which appeared through his pants. The women were amazed.

"This is for what?" they wanted to know.

"This is to merge us together," Coyote said. "I will show you."

"Is it necessary to put this in some part of my body?"

"Come over here, I will show you."

Coyote had sex with the two chief women, but other women in the village heard the sounds of joy and came running over, wanting some as well. Coyote had intercourse after intercourse, but eventually his cock went flat and shriveled up. The women who had not had sex began to paw at it to make it come back alive.

Coyote warned them that they'd get pregnant and have boys and girls, and the boys would have penises, but the women didn't believe him. They wanted sex! Coyote said he had to go pee first, but that no one was allowed to see him urinate, that it was against all the rules. And then Coyote ran to a canoe and paddled far away, leaving the women of the village behind.[6]

Here, the driving force of male prowess and domination is seen as something less efficient than male fantasy would like to believe, and Trickster is forced to retreat. The age-old mammalian pattern of male dominance to mate with as many females as possible is the ancient wiring on which the much more recent pair-bonding arrangements are built. Evolution always builds upon older structures, never makes them anew, so we live with these vestiges in our bodies and brains. But the male's dream of unlimited intercourse turns into a nightmare (which probably is a cautionary statement embedded in this tale—letting the lower, more primitive brain have its way does not lead to happiness). The story also shows women enjoying sex, and indeed evolution endowed them with genitalia to do just that: have orgasms. As theory predicts, there has to be no conscious awareness of why we do things, for evolution programs behaviors to reproduce our genes. The women here have no notion of pregnancy, yet they still have desire for sex. Ironically, it is Trickster who understands that sex leads to babies, which he has no desire to be responsible for. The exact age of this story is unknown, but it certainly challenges hundreds of years of Western religious admonishment stating sex is only for procreation.

Coyote and His Anus (Nez Perce, North America)

Coyote was wandering by a large stream and decided to get some fish to eat, so he built a weir and called to the salmon, and one came. Coyote killed him with a stick, made a fire, put on the salmon, and took a little snooze.

Racoon and Fox came along, saw Coyote asleep, and they decided to take the salmon and in its place put Coyote's anus, which they did by cutting it out of his rectum.

Coyote woke up, saw the salmon gone and immediately thought of Fox. But there was another good piece of scrumptious-looking meat on the fire, so Coyote ate it.

Then Fox and Racoon began to make a ruckus shouting, "It's your very own anus that you eat!"

Coyote reached behind him, and his anus was gone! He put the little piece of meat that he had not eaten back in place, but he had to keep his cheeks scrunched together when he walked to keep it in. Now he wanted revenge. He found Racoon and Fox sleeping later on and ate all the eggs they were cooking in the fire. Afterwards, though, Coyote and Fox had a good laugh, for they were very good friends.[7]

Here we have two tricksters, Coyote and Fox. Stories of bodily parts and functions are rampant in trickster tales, and there are numerous stories of Coyote devouring himself, particularily his anus. These stories comically portray a brain in conflict with itself and with the body in which it abides. Not exactly a Cartesian split between mind/body–reason/emotion, instead we see evidence of a division that goes something like this: mind/emotion/reason–body. Anything having to do with feces is disgusting in all cultures; in terms of a hierarchy of values it is at the bottom: waste.

The Trickster Myth Excerpts (Winnebago, North America)

In the Winnegabo Myth, the warriors were astonished to find Coyote having intercourse with a woman, which was a severe taboo before going to war. In this tale he burns his own anus and eats his own intestines. He puts his erect penis in a box and carries it on his back, only to send it out, snake-like, across the lake to enter the chief's daughter, until an old woman realizes what is happening and gets on top of the penis and pierces it with an awl, over and over again, for which Coyote says, "Why is she taking away all the fun?"[8]

Here in the second story, we have another anus and another penis out of control with Trickster eating his own intestines. One of the things trickster stories often address is ethics. Trickster often breaks the ethical taboos of the culture, showing the split between nature and nurture. Trickster has these tremendous appetites and urges given him by nature, which culture tries to reign in. Yet, the fact that universal taboos exist worldwide shows that ethics essentially derive from our universal biological selves, as Darwin originally proposed. In this story Trickster is so conflicted that he can even cannibalize himself without realizing it. Like us, Trickster is a creature more of emotion than logic. The neocortex is in control of nothing in most Trickster tales as the lower brain acts out its impulses. The humor of the story comes from that lack of control in the context of the underlying tension everyone knows exists. For one has to be in control in a human society, emotionally and physically in control of ourselves, even of our own flatulence. These stories point to the fact that, as Damasio says, "We are feeling machines that think, not thinking machines that feel." Trying to keep a lid on our most primal urges is a constant process with which the brain struggles.

Uncle Tompa (Tibet)

Uncle Tompa was a master weaver of wool, and it was customary for Tibetans to invite one such as this into their house, which is how Uncle Tompa ended up at the house of a mother and her daughter. The girl was a virgin and beautiful, and Uncle Tompa had tried for a few days to lure her into having sex with him, but to no avail. But then a plan came to him. He sat at his loom, and as the girl went downstairs to use the toilet, Uncle began working fervishly at his weaving. "Why are you doing that?" she asked.

Uncle Tompa said, "I too have to go to the bathroom, but I can't go until I finish this weave! But as you are going to the bathroom yourself, could you be kind enough to take my pee with you and deposit it in the toilet?"

The girl thought that would be fine, so Uncle Tompa had her undress, and he inserted his penis into her vagina and began having sex with her. The girl then went to the bathroom with Uncle's urine in her. But when she got back to the kitchen, she told her mother, who went through the roof. "No one can carry another's urine for them," she screamed. "He just had sex with you, is what he did!"

The girl got mad and went to the old man and yelled at him. "You screwed me," she said.

"No, I did not," said Uncle Tompa, "but if this is a problem, just let me have my urine back." So the girl let him take it out of her the same way he had put it in, taking her clothes off as he mounted her, having intercourse with the beautiful young girl again.[9]

This Tibetan trickster, like most tricksters, shows the unabashed power of evolution's most potent drive: to spread one's genes. For males, this means having as much sex as possible, but the female's interests are ignored, as without a pair-bond, she will be the one responsible (like most other mammals) to care for the offspring, while the man escapes responsibility. The disparity between male and female interests is the basis of everything from tribal gossip, to the novels of Jane Austen, to any soap opera on TV. Sexual proscriptions are put in place in every culture in the world to try and mitigate the possibility of a pregnancy that will not be legitimate (legitimacy equaling the degree of responsibility the male has to the female and the child). Trickster operates outside ethical boundaries, but his behavior also reveals the unbridled sexual drive of men. So on the one hand, these stories can act as cautionary tales to women, but at the same time they acknowledge that a kind of game is being played, and when Trickster outwits the young girl the audience would most likely laugh at his wit instead of admonishing him for his deceit.

Namaranganin (Aborigine, Australia)

The sisters, Jalmarida and Baiangun, from Dalingur, by Arnhem Bay, lived in the Dreaming. Cycad palm nuts they picked to stuff their dilly bags, which had to be dried in sunlight before they could be pounded into mash and made into a meal. As they waited for the nuts to dry, the two girls walked over to a mangrove swamp to find periwinkles from the mangrove roots.

Namaranganin resided in that place. He saw the two sisters and stalked them. Namaranganin made it rain in order to try and procure one of the girls, but the sisters recognized right away what was happening and began to run back to camp. Namaranganin jumped from out behind a tree and grabbed the younger sister, but the older one, Baiangun, got away. "Jalmarida, the younger one, she will be my wife," he said, and he picked her up and carried her into the jungle, but the older sister, Baiangun, ran back to the main camp and told what had happened, "Namaranganin took Jalmarida to the jungle . . . Namaranganin, the Trickster, who has the long erect member!" The men ran into the jungle to save Jalmarida.

Namaranganin, the Trickster, put Jalmarida in a hut that had a smoking fire. "Why can't the smoke escape?" Jalmarida asked, choking from it. Namaranganin said, "Because I want to have sex with you." But Jalmarida said, "No, you can't do it, because Dagurura is inside my vagina." (Dagurura is a stone and a totemic emblem.) Namaranganin took a sharp stick and got out the stone from her vagina, but then a sound began roaring and the sacred Wonguri totemic water burst out as the stone moved along the water as Namaranganin sang. (Taking the stone out made sex easier for human women).

The village men found Namaranganin and ran spears through him and burnt him in a bonfire. But Jalmarida did not go back home with the villagers. She made herself into a fly.[10]

Coyote Sleeps with His Own Daughters
(Southern Ute, North America)

Coyote was a father with a son and two daughters. As he lay on his blanket, he saw that the ceiling was leaking, so he commanded one of his daughters to stop the leak. As she went up the ladder, he saw her vulva and got very hot, and his penis grew big. So he told the other daughter to do the same so he could see her vulva. She climbed the ladder as well. "This is a taboo," he said to himself, yet he still thought that was something he could get around. He had no more interest in his wife, who was old. He picked up something sharp and made his chest bleed, yelling to his wife that he was dying from an enemy who had entered their lodge. He then told the family to burn his body on a funeral pyre when he was gone and to move to another village to make a new life, but not to look once the fire had been lit. So Coyote pretended he was dead, and the wife and two daughters wrapped him in his blanket, put it on the funeral pyre and ignited it. But the little boy disobeyed, looked, and saw his father, Coyote, slip from the blanket and get away. He told his mother and sisters, but no one believed the little boy.

They moved to a new village, and it didn't take long before a handsome young man came to call, riding a fine horse, and he was dressed to the hilt in rich otter skins as well. Of course, it was Coyote, who can shape-shift into anything. The girls wanted to marry the good-looking young man, and their mother thought that would be good as well, but the little boy yelled that this young man looked like their father, Old Man Coyote! The mother and daughters thought the little boy was nuts.

So Coyote married the daughters, and he took the first daughter to bed that night and had sex with her, very much liking the fact that she was young and tender, unlike his old wife. Then Coyote asked the little boy to go fetch him a rabbit to eat, which was something the little boy knew was what his father always had done. He proved that the young husband really was Old Man Coyote by pointing out four missing teeth, which Coyote had not been able to make new when he shape-shifted. Once Coyote's wife realized what was going on she grabbed a butcher knife and went after Coyote, who said, "Ok, ok, I'll just sleep with you, wife, from now on." But the sisters were shamed, flung themselves into the night sky and turned to stars.[11]

Here, Coyote has his way with his two daughters, violating the incest taboo, which is universal to human cultures, and no doubt has a biological origin to prevent genetic problems that can stem from inbreeding. Darwin believed that evolution had programmed animals to avoid inbreeding, as inbreeding may cause more harmful mutations in offspring. This was debated for many years. Edward Westermarck laid out the biological imperatives for incest avoidance in his book *The History of Human Marriage* (first published in 1889, which were in direct contrast to Freud's belief that incest was a common desire in humans and only culture could put it at bay). The evidence has come clearly down on the side of Westermarck, for primate studies have shown that it is very unlikely that primates raised together to ever desire to mate. In addition, in the wild, chimp females leave their original troops and move elsewhere. In baboons it is the males who leave. In human societies, siblings who have been raised together have a strong aversion to mating. Incest does occur in humans, but all the evidence supports a biological root for the incest taboo, which customs and laws in every culture amplify.

How Kwaku Ananse Got Aso in Marriage (Ashanti, Africa)

There once lived a certain man called Akwasi-the-jealous-one, and his wife was Aso. His wife was Aso, and he did not want anyone to see Aso or anyone to talk to to her. So he went and built a small settlement for Aso to live in. Now Akwasi-the-jealous-one could not beget children. Because of that, if he and his wife lived in town, someone would take her away.

Sky-god told the young men, "Akwasi-the-jealous-one has been married to Aso for a very, very long time. She has not conceived by him and borne a child. Therefore, he who is able, let him go and take Aso and, should she conceive by him, let him take her as his wife."

All the young men tried their best to lay hands on her, but not one was able.

Now Kwaku Ananse [the spider], was there watching these events, and he said, "I can go to Akwasi-the- jealous-one's village."

Sky-god said, "Can you really do so?"

Ananse said, "If you will give me what I require."

Sky-god said, "What kind of thing?"

He said, "Medicine for gun and bullets."

And the sky-god gave it to him. Ananse took the powder and bullets to various small villages, saying, "Sky-god has bade me to bring powder and bullets to you, and you are to go and kill meat. On the day I shall return here, I shall take the meat and depart." He distributed the powder and the bullets among very many small villages, until all were finished. All the villagers got him some meat.

On a certain day Ananse wove a palm-leaf basket. Its length was from here to over yonder. Ananse took it to the small villages where he had distributed the powder and bullets to receive all the meat which they had killed. Father Ananse took the meat and palm-leaf basket, set them on his head, and set out on the path leading to Akwasi-the-jealous-one's settlement. When he reached the stream from which Akwasi and his wife drank, he picked out some meat and put it in. Ananse strode hard and brought the palm-leaf basket full of meat and passed through the main entrance leading into Akwasi-the-jealous-one's compound.

Aso saw him. She said, "Akwasi!! Come and look at something which is coming to the house here. What can it be?"

Ananse said, "It is the Sky-god who is sending me. I am weary, and I am coming to sleep here."

Akwasi-the-jealous-one said, "I have heard my lord's servant."

Aso said to Ananse, "Father man, some of your meat has fallen down at the main entrance to the compound."

The spider said, "Oh, if you happen to have a dog, let him go and take that meat and chew on it."

So Aso went and got it and gave it to her husband.

Then Ananse said, "Mother, set some food on the fire for me."

Aso put some on, and Ananse said, "Mother, is it fufuo that you are cooking or eto?"

Aso replied, "Fufuo."

Ananse said, "Then it is too little; go and fetch a big pot."

Aso went and fetched a big one.

Ananse said, "Come and get meat." There were forty hindquarters of great beasts. He said, "Take these only and put them in. "If you had a pot big enough, I would give you enough meat to chew to make your teeth fall out."

Aso finished preparing the food, turned it out of the pot, and placed it on a table, splashed water, and put it beside the rest of the food. Then Aso took her portion and went and set it down near the fire. And the men went and sat down beside the table. They touched the backs of each other's hands.

While they were eating, Kwaku Ananse said, "There is no salt in this fufuo."

Akwasi said to Aso, "Bring some salt."

But Ananse said, "Not at all. When the woman is eating, you tell her to get up to bring salt. You yourself should go and bring it."

Akwasi got up, and Ananse looked into his bag and took out a pinch of purgative medicine and put it in the fufuo.

Then he called Akwasi, saying, "Come back for I have brought some with me."

When Akwasi came Ananse said, "Oh, I shall eat no more. I am full."

Akwasi, who suspected nothing, continued eating.

When they had finished eating, Akwasi said, "Friend, we and you are sitting here, and yet we do not know your name."

Ananse said, "I am called Rise-up-and-make-love-to-Aso.'"

Akwasi said, "I have heard, and you, Aso, have you heard this man's name?"

Aso replied, "Yes, I have heard."

Akwasi rose to go and prepare one of the spare bedrooms and to make everything comfortable.

He said, "Rise-up-and-make-love-to-Aso, this is your room. Go and sleep there."

The spider said, "I am the soul-washer to Sky-god, and I sleep in an open veranda room. Since mother bore me and father begat me, I have never slept in a closed bedroom."

Akwasi said, "Then where will you sleep?"

He replied, "Were I to sleep in this open veranda room here, that would make you equal to Sky-god, for it would mean that I was sleeping in the Sky-god's open veranda room. Since I am never to sleep in any-one's open room except that of a Sky-god, I shall just lie down in front of this closed sleeping-room where you repose."

The man took out a sleeping mat and laid it there for him. Akwasi and his wife went to rest, and Ananse, too, lay down there. Ananse lay there

*and he slipped in the crossbar of the bedroom door. Ananse lay there
and took his musical bow and sang:*

> *"Akuamoa Ananse, today we shall achieve something, today.*
> *Ananse, the child of Nsia, the mother of Nyame, the sky-god,*
> *Today we shall achieve something, today.*
> *Ananse, the Soul-washer to Nyame, the sky-god,*
> *Today I shall see some–thing."*

*Now, he stopped playing his musical instrument and laid it aside, and
then he lay down.*

*He slept for some time when he heard Akwasi-the-jealous-one calling,
"Father man!"*

Not a sound in reply except the chirping of the cicada, dinn!

"Father man!"

Not a sound in reply except dinn!

*Akwasi-the- jealous-one was dying. The medicine had taken effect on
him, but he calls, "Father man!"*

Not a sound in reply except the chirping of the cicada, dinn!

At last he said, "Rise-Up-and–make-love-to-Aso! "

The spider said, "Mm! Mm! Mm!"

Akwasi said, "Open the door for me."

Ananse opened the door, and Akwasi went somewhere.

And the spider rose up and went into the room there.

He said, "Aso, did you not hear what your husband said?"

She replied, "What did he say?"

Ananse replied, "He said I must rise up and make love to you."

Aso said, "You don't lie."

And he did it for her, and he went and lay down.

*That night Akwasi rose up nine times. The spider also went nine times
to where Aso was.*

When things became visible next morning, Ananse went off.

It would be about two moons later when Aso's belly became large.

*Akwasi questioned her, saying, "Why has your belly got like this? Per-
haps you are ill, for you know that I who live with you here am unable
to beget children."*

*Aso replied, "You forget that man who came here whom you told to rise
up and make love to Aso. Well, he took me and I have conceived by him."*

Akwasi-the-jealous-one said, "Rise up, and let me take you to go and give you to him." They went to Sky-god's town. On the way Aso gave birth.

They reached Sky-god's town and Akwasi went and told Sky-god what had happened, saying, "A subject of yours, whom you sent, slept at my house and took Aso, and she conceived by him."

Sky-god said, "All of my subjects are roofing the houses: go and point out the one you mean."

They went off, and the spider was sitting on a ridge–pole.

Aso said, "There he is!"

And Ananse ran and sat on the middle.

Again Aso said, "There he is!"

Then Ananse fell down from where he was sitting.

Now that day was Friday.

Ananse said, "I, who was Sky-god's soul—you have taken your hand and pointed it at me, so that I have fallen down and got red earth on me."

Immediately, the attendants seized hold of Akwasi-the-jealous-one and made him sacrifice a sheep. When Akwasi-the-jealous-one had fin- ished sacrificing the sheep, he said to Sky-god, "Here is the woman; let Ananse take her."

So Ananse took Aso, but as for the infant, they killed it, cut it into pieces, and scattered them about.

That is how jealousy came among the tribe.

This, my story, which I have related, if it be sweet, or if it be not sweet, some you may take as true, and the rest you may praise me for telling of it.[12]

Emotions control our thoughts, often determine our ethical choices, and make us who we are. There is no such thing as pure logic, for with- out emotion we could not make even the most basic decisions (which Damasio has shown). Jealousy is an emotion that relates directly to the pair-bonding, which developed in our species probably some 200,000 years ago. Much is at stake in a marriage situation, and evolution has developed strong emotional bonds to keep couples together. When these bonds are threatened, violence can erupt, and domestic violence accounts for a huge percentage of violence around the world, with somewhere near six times more of it directed at women by men than men by women. In this trickster story we see the age-old notion of marriage as "ownership" played out, stemming from the ancient problem of paternity in human relations. The male wants to ensure that *his* DNA is what is being reproduced by his wife's pregnancy.

But there is also the case of being "barren" in this story, as obviously the old man is infertile, and the people in the tribe are quite aware of this. Being barren puts the tribe in danger, as every child is precious. Many children will die young, and survival of the culture is always at risk. The sky-god is aware of this too and allows any man who can make Aso conceive to have her as his wife. Aso herself seems to have little control of her own destiny, being manipulated by her husband, the tribe, and the sky-god. Yet, fertility is the key to evolutionary success, and this ethical perspective trumps the marriage vows. Trickster, of course, tries to remedy the situation, and does the job. But there is a price to be paid for violating the pair-bond marriage relationship. For Jealousy is unleashed upon the world, due to the violations by Trickster, which sky-god himself condones. Instead of new life for the tribe, who themselves become murderers, there is death, and now Jealousy threatens the entire community forever.

Coyote Keeps His Dead Wife's Genitals
(Lipan Apache, North America)

Coyote's wife died. Before he disposed of her body, he cut her genitals off, and after that he dried them and pounded them to a powder, which he put in a pouch. Every time he got lonely for his wife, he took this package out and sprinkled some of the powder on his penis. It caused an orgasm every time.

Coyote had several sons. They saw their father go away by himself with his pouch several times. They snooped around and finally saw what he was doing. One time when he was away they stole his pouch. They stood around and sprinkled the powder on their penises. It caused erections and orgasms, and they were ejaculating in all directions.

Just then Coyote came in and found them at it. He was very angry. He scolded them and beat them. "It was just for myself," he said. "You had no business taking it. Which of you did it work on?" "It didn't work on me," the smallest son said. "No white stuff came out, though my penis grew big. I had only a pouch."[13]

There are many stories of Trickster longing for his dead wife. Here we see that even after death the lust for a wife remains, even when her genitals are ground up into a powder. Much has been written about women's ability to create new life in contrast to the lesser role played by men, and how ultimately the power of men is limited. Even though Trickster can have an orgasm it cannot lead to anything. No new life is being formed. But once again, even in a futile situation, nature has programmed the brain for sex regardless of an outcome, for the process of evolution demands that an organism does not have to be aware of why it acts the way it does.

⑬

FEMALE TRICKSTERS

A man's face is his autobiography. A woman's face is her fiction.

—Oscar Wilde

While the majority of trickster figures around the world are male, for which reason I have primarily used "he" instead of "she" in describing trickster characters, there *are* female tricksters as well as tricksters who can shape-shift from male to female through a transsexual or transgender slight of hand. Then again, there are tricksters who are hermaphrodites. Esu, a trickster of the Yorbu of Western Africa, is often portrayed in statuary as paired—both male and female—or as a single bisexual figure—even though he performs tremendous feats with his notorious penis, he/she is also often holding her prominent breasts:

> Certainly [Esu] is not restricted to human distinctions of gender or sex; he is at once both male and female. Although his masculinity is depicted as visually and graphically overwhelming, his equally expressive femininity renders his enormous sexuality ambiguous, contrary, and genderless.[1]

As remarkable and powerful as these bisexual manifestations of Esu are, it is too often the case that when it comes to the female tricksters they are portrayed as being devious and manipulative, reflecting the misogyny of cultures the world over which give preference to the male and cast women as second-class citizens: in the case of state-level societies we see women often reduced to chattel. Trickster literature is littered with stereotypical witches, temptresses, sexual predators, and whores: women who use evil cunning and subtle wiles to manipulate and control men. On the other hand, as in all stories, interpretation is key to meaning, and even in stories where dominant men control women there is often the hint of inherent feminine power at the core of these tales— power that men find dangerous and threatening. When told by men, this power is seen as ominous, but looked at in another light such stories not only reveal the hysterical fear men can have regarding powerful women, but the very fact that women are not the "weaker sex."

The first known historical folk tale of a female trickster is "The Two Brothers," from Egypt of the thirteenth-century BC (This story, of course, comes from a state-level society, not a tribal culture). In this story, the Queen attempts to seduce her brother-in-law, who rebukes her. She then lies to her husband, telling him that his brother has tried to engage her in a sexual liaison. The King is inflamed and murders his brother. The nearly identical story is played out in the biblical story of Joseph, where Joseph is seduced by Joseph's master's wife—Potiphar— from Genesis 3.9:

[7] And it came to pass after these things, that his master's wife cast her eyes upon Joseph; and she said, Lie with me.
[8] But he refused, and said unto his master's wife, Behold, my master wotteth not what is with me in the house, and he hath committed all that he hath to my hand;
[9] There is none greater in this house than I; neither hath he kept back any thing from me but thee, because thou art his wife: how then can I do this great wickedness, and sin against God?
[10] And it came to pass, as she spake to Joseph day by day, that he hearkened not unto her, to lie by her, or to be with her.
[11] And it came to pass about this time, that Joseph went into the house to do his business; and there was none of the men of the house there within.
[12] And she caught him by his garment, saying, Lie with me: and he left his garment in her hand, and fled, and got him out.

[13] And it came to pass, when she saw that he had left his garment in her hand, and was fled forth,

[14] That she called unto the men of her house, and spake unto them, saying, See, he hath brought in an Hebrew unto us to mock us; he came in unto me to lie with me, and I cried with a loud voice:

[15] And it came to pass, when he heard that I lifted up my voice and cried, that he left his garment with me, and fled, and got him out.

[16] And she laid up his garment by her, until his lord came home.

[17] And she spake unto him according to these words, saying, The Hebrew servant, which thou hast brought unto us, came in unto me to mock me:

[18] And it came to pass, as I lifted up my voice and cried, that he left his garment with me, and fled out.

[19] And it came to pass, when his master heard the words of his wife, which she spake unto him, saying, After this manner did thy servant to me; that his wrath was kindled.

[20] And Joseph's master took him, and put him into the prison, a place where the king's prisoners were bound: and he was there in the prison.

[21] But the LORD was with Joseph, and shewed him mercy, and gave him favour in the sight of the keeper of the prison.

Tales of dangerous seductresses occur worldwide, where the woman entices a man and brings about his downfall. They occur in tribal as well as state-level societies, so this theme is very ancient and certainly reflects fears of responsibility on the part of the male. For unlike chimps and bonobos, the human male is required by the biology of the pair-bond (and the corresponding terms of society—marriage) to give of himself to his mate and offspring. Here we see how this newer disposition, fueled by evolution, toward monogamy/pair-bonding/marriage conflicts with the much older case of promiscuity in our species. Of course questions of paternity are always paramount in the minds of men (as mentioned previously), so control of women's reproduction has been an insane obsession. This is why virginity has traditionally been seen as universally important across human cultures—so a man is secure in the knowledge that no other male DNA has entered "his" woman before he has penetrated her. But men do not just have sex with their wives. The double standard is pernicious: it's all right for a man to sleep with as many women as he wishes, while the woman is supposed to remain chaste.

Of course, this is mathematically impossible, and some women who (for whatever reason) were not married, took sexual partners for pay, or for love—giving up any claim to virginity—while often ruining their chances for matrimony and/or ruining their reputations in the community. The male, often on the prowl for more sexual partners, could easily find himself in a dalliance with such a woman (a non-virgin), become amorous and then find himself in a position of becoming a father. (As we have seen, evolution programs us to act in certain ways that have nothing to do with logic—contrary to the Catholic Church's stance procreation is often the farthest thing from our minds as we engage in sex). Even though women are of the utmost value to men in tribal cultures, and are often a reason for warfare (to capture more women), evolution has left our species with a legacy of the double standard where women have typically been seen as either the Madonna or the Whore. It's important to realize that even though such mindsets are tied to our biological evolution, that does not mean society is incapable of overriding such dispositions. The importance of virginity in the West has declined to the point of nearly zero, due to birth control, the Women's Movement, and societal views on sex, even though it lives on in many places in India, Africa, and Asia. Yet, at the same time, the old double standard has not abated. Men still worry about entrapment from women, and men who are promiscuous are never seen as sluts or whores. They are studs.

The first time I heard a Vagina Dentate story was while visiting a medicine man friend on the Pine Ridge Indian Reservation, back in the early 1970s. Selo Black Crow was a "holy man" of the Ogallala Sioux. He related a story to a group of us one afternoon as we were looking out over his 800 acres scattered with buffalo, just a few miles east of Wanblee, South Dakota. Selo said his mother had told him this story when he was a child—that there are women who have teeth in their vaginas, and that because of this a man should always be on the watch for such women, and all women in general, for you could never know when a female might be one of these and get you—gnawing off your penis when you went inside of her.

Little did I know at the time, this is a myth that has occurred in a variety of cultures around the world (not made up by Freud, as some believe, though he made reference to it). In a similar vein, years earlier, as a fourteen-year-old working in the cornfields of Illinois, detasseling corn, I heard a story from our team leader who had been to Vietnam. He told us that the Vietnamese women prostitutes would often insert razor blades into their vaginas to shred the penises of American soldiers. Though complete myth, it was an image that scared the hell out of us young boys working our way through the flatlands of Illinois. These are both trickster stories, to be sure, but here the female Trickstar is cruel and evil, with nothing of the enchanting, comic quality found in so many of the male trickster tales.

There are a host of stories that paint women as tricksters of this type—with women being portrayed in a hideous fashion. And of course, there are numerous taboos in cultures around the world where menstruating women are seen as evil or dangerous (I have come across this belief many times, even in tribal people today). Sometimes, the fact that women must be put away from the tribe in separate huts has undergone a revisionist interpretation as a "sacred" time for the woman, but a closer look at the ethnographic literature shows that it is male fear of women's blood that initiates these practices and that there is a negative connotation to menstruation. The traditional interpretation given by anthropologists and folklorists in the past (such as Campbell), that primal men somehow feared (or were jealous of) the life-giving abilities of women may or may not be true. But for many cultures, blood is considered "life," hence the worldwide fascination with sacrifice and blood-letting, for animals, or humans. Recall that Cain killed Abel because God was not satisfied with Cain's sacrifice of grain. It had to be blood. I am inclined to believe that it is fear of blood itself, coming from the reproductive area of women's bodies that frightened men. It was unexplainable, and did not seem to be natural, in that it was not observed in other animals. It was seen as powerful, but usually an evil power.

Some female trickster stories that appear negative can be reinterpreted through a feminist critique that makes the villain the heroine. A reinterpretation of Eve as culture hero is such an example. She becomes the one who brings enlightenment and consciousness to humanity, instead of the evildoer, seducing mankind into a life of misery. (Such an interpretation was actually conceived by early Christian Gnostics nearly 2,000 years ago. However, such interpretations are far and away historically rare [or hidden] in our society. Indeed, many of those Gnostic texts that were sympathetic to women were burned by the soldiers of the newly Christianized Roman Empire.)

Marilyn Jurich, in her seminal study of female tricksters, *Scheherazade's Sisters*, asks why the woman/devil connection is so prominent: "Are women then, even more unscrupulous and malicious than this very archetype of evil? [Does this] mean that women are by nature diabolical or, at least, tainted?"[2] The Old Testament presents a raft of other "evil" women: Delilah, who cut Samson's hair and took away his power. Then there were Lot's virgin daughters, and his wife. Lot had offered his daughters up to the men of Sodom to rape instead of sodomizing the male ambassadors from God whom Lot had been hosting. But the people declined. As the daughters are escaping, with their mother and father, from God's wrath at the evil of the city, Lot's wife is turned into a pillar of salt because she disobeyed God's command by looking back at the sacked and burning city. Later Lot's daughters trick their father into having sex with them in order to perpetuate the human species, by violating the incest taboo. The moral of the story shows them to be damned.

Cultures around the world reiterate this theme of bad women (for all the underlying reasons we have seen). But this is not always the case. Going against the grain, the biblical story of Tabor is one in which craftiness on the part of a woman pays off. Tabor, a widow, tricks her father-in-law into impregnating her, thereby securing her future, though she takes her life into her own hands by this action—for a man was allowed to sleep with as many prostitutes as he desired—but a woman accused of sexual misconduct could be burned at the stake.

The tale of Scheherazade is the most famous case of all where a woman is able to turn the tables and on a man. This story is the frame which begins *The Arabian Nights*, and it is a story of cunning and survival in which Scheherazade outsmarts the King and saves her own head, as well as the heads of many other women in the kingdom.

Both wives of King Shahzaman and his brother are found to have secret lovers, so the wives and their lovers are executed. Thinking that all women are evil, the two brothers plot revenge upon womankind, especially the young maidens who are of age to marry. A new bride is brought to the King each night, but after having sexual relations with her, each bride is executed the following morning. This goes on and on, until Scheherazade bravely asks to be the next bride. But she has hatched a plan with her sister, Dinarzad. After the King has sex with Scheherazade, Scheherazade's sister, Dinarzad, enters the chamber and suggests that Scheherazade tell the King a story before her death. So Scheherazade begins telling the stories of *The Arabian Nights*, carefully crafting each tale so that the King is left in suspense evening after evening, for a thousand nights, until the King falls in love with Scheherazade, eventually marrying her, and together they have three children. Not only does Scheherazade end up in the most prestigious position in the kingdom, she saves the lives of countless other women through her act of sacrifice and stealth. As Marilyn Jurich says in *Scheherazade's Sisters*:

> To understand what constitutes the "tricks of women," it is necessary to look at the *trick* itself. The trick by its very nature is left (sinister or devious), underhanded, rather than right (straight or direct), truthful, on the level. Its natural connection, then, seems to be with the diabolical, for evil is dark and secret and takes us unprepared. The trick works because it is covert and often contrary to what we anticipate. . . . Tricks and women form a natural association; both have been traditionally suspect, regarded with a mixture of suspicion and awe, and both depend on cunning and indirection. The notion of a woman playing tricks, then, compounds our fascination, even as it confirms our expectation. The nature of trickster, then, is substantially intensified in the dealings of the woman trickster, the *trickstar*. Sometimes her artifices shock us, motivated as they are by malice and self-interest. At other times, her caprices amuse; and we admire her ability to contrive her way out of confining, even life-threatening circumstances, and respect her determination to seek social justice for others. Tradition, however—that tradition supported by male power—often prefers to see the trickstar as menacing, her tricks as self-serving.[3]

Franchot Ballinger, in "Coyote, He/She Was Going There: Sex and Gender in Native American Trickster Stories," also asks the question of why there are so few female tricksters. He goes through a possible litany of reasons—that anthropologists tended to speak with male informants, that EuroAmerican attitudes toward female tricksters would have prevented publication of female trickster stories, that in primal societies gender for trickster didn't matter, *or* he asks whether it is the case that in patralineal cultures Tricksters are mostly male and that in matrilineal cultures they are mostly female. But none of these questions are convincing, with little evidence for justifying them. In matrilineal Pueblo cultures of the Southwest United States, Trickster is male in the form of Coyote, even if the Coyote story is told by a woman. All of these theories are strained, and while possibly true in a few instances, they cannot answer the larger question of Trickster's maleness. Ballinger goes on to state that

> in the few female trickster stories available to us, she is commonly the object of the satire. The questions arise: Is she satirized because she is a woman or is she satirized because she is a trickster who incidentally is female? What, if any, relationship exists between the trickster's gender and the narrative elements in the stories? I believe that in most female trickster stories the protagonist's trickster personality causes her to fall short of her community's gender role expectations. She is, therefore, fair game for satire, as is the male trickster personality when he fails his society's expectations, some of them gender-related, for example, when he fails both as a warrior and a chief in the Winnebago cycle or when he perverts his father's role by marrying his daughter.[4]

Tales in which female tricksters are fallen women are obviously based upon cultural rules regarding what is required of women, but in addition, as Lori Landy says in *Madcaps, Screwballs, and Con Women*— tricksterism can also be a matter of opportunity.

> In a sexist society, the male trickster clearly has the advantages of masculinity: mobility, autonomy, power, and safety. He is able to be a liminal figure who can move between the margins and centers of society as he deconstructs the power systems with his humor and trickery. In fact, his experiences in female form are often a period of stability, which he leaves behind to continue on his adventures. He performs his tactical ridicule in the public sphere, mocking and subverting the existing political, social, and economic structures. Obviously, women have not had the same opportunities for such a high degree of mobility (physical as well as psychological, social, economic, artistic, and political). Thus when scholars have looked for trickster figures using definitions based on the assumptions of the trickster's masculinity, they haven't found female figures who fit. In order to identify female tricksters in American (or any) culture, therefore, we must turn from the margins of dominant society to the centers of women's space—the parlors, kitchens, and bedrooms of domesticity.[5]

When it comes to discovering living and mythic tricksters, Landay is right, that we have to look in new environments to discover new cases of Trickstars, but that argument only goes so far. Men certainly have had the advantages of mobility and visibility, but this explanation misses one of the central points of Trickster—that he generates humor. The main reason trickster tales are about male figures is that the testosterone-driven male, consumed with thoughts of sexual adventure and hierarchical dominance, who is willing to take great risks to satisfy his urges, creates a far more comical, outlandish character. Trickster tales most often revolve around desire and frustration. It is the male's more pronounced reaching out (with his penis, his hands, or his inflated ego, or his drive to be top banana) that allows for the foil. His big ambitions make for a much greater fall. The male trickster is the fool because of his cravings for status, power, sex, food, and hedonistic pleasure; and trickster tales often infer the absurdity and shortsightedness of these desires—the senselessness of self-aggrandizement and the constant struggle for hierarchical dominance—which the Trickster often both symbolizes and mocks. When the comedy rests upon the quest for personal satisfaction, men seem to naturally have a lot more pretensions for stories to reveal, hence having greater comedic value. Comedy can only occur when there is a disconnect. There must be an imbalance for which laughter is the remedy. The tale, and the laughter that ensues, is in a sense an exorcism, the germ of which can be found in cultures around the world who believe that stories, narratives, confessions, songs, through the act of being told, also heal. Trickster stories often revolve around disparities between men and women. Humor is what society needs in the face of adversity. The pomposity of the male needs to be kept in check, for in the end both males and females must get along.

From a feminist perspective, the male trickster can be seen as the ultimate nightmare, the supreme sexist pig, and the epitome of hedonistic masculinity. But the fact that he is brought out in the open and laughed at takes him down to size. Women in tribal cultures are usually not shielded from trickster stories. On the contrary, women often take delight in these tales as much as men. But when there are stories of women tricksters (Trickstars), they often reflect another side of biology and culture as Ballinger suggests. Another dynamic is at work, in which the raucous laughter emitted from hearing the male's stories, is absent. For the rules governing women's behavior, when it comes to sexuality, marriage, and childbirth, are enmeshed in the double standard, and women have traditionally been caught in the snare of duplicitous regulation. So it follows that the female trickster would be confronting a whole other set of constraints imposed upon her than those imposed upon men (no matter whether the societies are patralineal or matrilineal). A different kind of humor emerges when a woman is the Trickstar protagonist, especially when the outcome for her is good. There are women tricksters who rise above oppression and enduring stereotypes, showing that women can be just as wily as men, just as smart, just as clever, and just as much in control—even when the world surrounding them is brutal and constantly against them. As a matter of fact, living in a world that has historically been dominated by men, one aspect of Trickster—antithesis of the status-quo—would seem most naturally to belong to women. For Trickster is notorious for challenging hierarchy. Trickster is the original rebel. To the male, being tamed can mean being wed, being responsible for a family, or being subservient in society. To the female, the dangers she must confront include being pregnant without a mate, being locked in a loveless marriage, and/or forced into servitude. Since she often has the force of tradition downgrading her because she is a woman, the female Trickstar must utilize alternative ways to achieve her own desires for freedom, when any kind of overt action is impossible. Maybe Ballinger is right, that there are more female trickster stories out there than we know—they are just hidden. Or maybe women advertising their real abilities in a trickster story would have not been as productive for them, as women, until recently, were often forced to wear the trickster mask in real life, a mask that said *we are oblivious to the machinations of men.* Some of the female trickster stories show this—the essential power and intelligence of women, their tenacity to survive the misogyny of male-dominated cultures that have controlled them and coerced them into stereotypes. In the story from India, we see that when women want to assert their intelligence they disguise themselves as men. Such folk legends found their way into numerous plots of Shakespeare's plays, where women prove themselves smarter than the men who wish to control, dominate, or wed them.

EVIL WOMAN TRICKSTER STORIES

The Toothed Vagina (Yurok, North America)

Coyote was wandering along when he noticed two girls harvesting hazelnuts. They had a guy with him they both liked, Cotton Tail Rabbit.

Coyote asked where they were spending the night and if he could camp with them, so they told him and said "ok."

The sandbar in the river is where they camped. Rabbit slept at the girl's feet, while Coyote got right between them, sharing a blanket, always pulling the blanket to just cover himself and complaining that the girls' breasts were too big.

The girls hated Coyote and felt sorry for their friend Rabbit, so the three of them decided to get away from Coyote as fast as possible.

Rabbit said, "All right," and they put logs on both sides of Coyote so he would think they were still there, and went across the river and stayed.

Coyote was really mad, but Rabbit, wanting the girls for himself, sent a trick that made Coyote drown, so he was nothing but bones. Coyote was really pissed. He came to a camp where there were kids, and he thought they all had to be Rabbit's, so he set a fire and burned them all up. Then he heard a story. Apparently, there was a lady upriver who killed every man who slept with her through intercourse, because she had teeth inside her vagina. Outside her tepee was a yard full of bones.

As soon as Coyote saw this woman he wanted to have sex with her, but he gathered a bundle of sticks, and instead of his penis, he put one stick inside her instead. That stick was gnawed down to nothing so Coyote put another into her vagina. He did this ten times, but the woman couldn't take this many times of having intercourse and died.

Coyote had "cured" this problem, saying, "From that time on Coyote made it safe for men to have sex with women.[6]

Teeth in the Wrong Place (Ponca-Otoe, North America)

Coyote was wandering when he heard of an old lady with two beautiful daughters. But if men tried to sleep with the daughters they were not heard from again. Coyote had to check this out, not believing it true.

When he got to the tepee, the old lady let him in and the two beautiful daughters fed him. People are crazy, Coyote said. These women are wonderful!

At nighttime the old lady put Coyote between the two girls to keep him warm. But the younger one whispered to him that she was not really a daughter of the old lady, who was a witch, but the other sister was the witch's daughter. She herself had been kidnapped. The older "sister" would come on to Coyote, the young girl said, but the witch mother had put teeth in both of the girls' vaginas in order to kill young men so the old witch could rob them of their goods. Coyote listened. He could hear the teeth in the girls' vaginas, grinding.

Soon, the older "sister" did just as the younger girl had said. "Have sex with me," she said to Coyote. But Coyote got a stick from the fire and put it in her vagina instead. Chips and wood slices soon began spitting out of her vagina. Then Coyote stuck an arrow into the girl and killed her, and then he killed the old lady witch in the same way.

Coyote told the younger girl he wanted to marry her, and they fled right away. Once they were far from that evil house, Coyote wanted to have sex with the girl. "But how?" she asked. "I have the same affliction! I have teeth in my vagina." So Coyote knocked the teeth out of her vagina with a stick, leaving just one, which give them both extra stimulation when they did it, making the two very happy indeed.[7]

Proverbs 5: 3–8 (Hebrew)

3: For the lips of a strange woman drop as an honeycomb, and her mouth is smoother than oil:

4: But her end is bitter as wormwood, sharp as a two-edged sword.

5: Her feet go down to death; her steps take hold on hell.

6: Lest thou shouldest ponder the path of life, her ways are moveable, that thou canst not know them.

7: Hear me now therefore, O ye children, and depart not from the words of my mouth.

8: Remove thy way far from her, and come not nigh the door of her house.

CLEVER/GOOD WOMEN TRICKSTER STORIES

Old Coyote Man Meets Coyote Woman
(Blackfoot, North America)

At the dawn of time there were only two beings, Old Coyote Man and Old Coyote Woman, and somehow they met, recognizing immediately that they were identical, except that Old Coyote Woman saw that Old Coyote Man had something. "What is it?" she asked.

In his sack was a penis.

Old Coyote looked in her sack, and there was a vagina.

"Let's put them into our navels," said Coyote Man, but Coyote Woman thought they best be placed between each of their legs, then they realized that they fit together, and they began to make love. After awhile, they thought this might be the way to make people, but how should they look? Old Coyote Man got it all wrong, thinking that eyes and mouth should be lined up long ways on the face, and that the women should obey the men. But Old Coyote Woman put things right, which is why people look the way they do today.[8]

The Most Precious Thing in the World (Hebrew)

After ten years of being childless, a man wanted to divorce his wife, even though he loved her, so he went to Rabbi Simeon ben Yohai, who tried to encourage the man to stay married, since he loved his wife, after all. But if nothing could fix this, he said they should have a feast to end the marriage, just as they had had a feast to begin their union. That way they could still part friends. This they had at a fine establishment in town, and at the feast, the wife made sure that her husband got drunk on wine. The husband said to her, before passing out, "Darling, procure the most precious things from our house before you leave."

The man passed out in a stupor, and the wife had him carried back to the house of his father by the other guests. When the man woke he was flabbergasted to find himself at the house he had grown up in. "What is going on?" he asked.

"I did what you asked," said the wife. "I took the most precious thing, which is you!"

The husband repented and nine months after that they had a son.[9]

The Wife Who Refused to Be Beaten (Kashmiri, India)

A wealthy mercantilist from Kashmir valley had a stupid son. The mercantilist hired the best tutors in the country, but the son was incapable of learning. He was lazy and wasted his time. The father began hating his son, but the boy's mother loved him.

When he was old enough to be married, the mother wanted to find a mate for her son, but the mercantilist was against it: his son was just too dumb to be married. Yet, it was shameful to have a child not get married, and the mother kept asking her husband to find the boy a mate. The mercantilist was fed up, but one day he relented, setting a task for the boy. He gave his son three pansas and told him to go down to the market and purchase food with one pansa, to toss another pansa into the river, and with the last pansa to procure these things—food, drink, a thing to chew, something to plant in the garden, and he was to buy food for the cow.

The boy went to the market and purchased some food with one pansa. He went next down to the river and was about to toss a pansa into it, when the idea of that seemed ridiculous. Why waste a pansa? Yet, he wanted to do as he'd been told. Just then the daughter of an ironsmith appeared and saw that he was upset. He explained to the girl what his dilemma was, but she had a plan.

"A watermelon contains all the five things, buy one and keep the other pansa in your pocket instead of throwing it into the river."

When he got home, the mercantilist's wife was very happy and told her husband how smart their son actually was, but the mercantilist thought someone must have coaxed the boy, for this was beyond his mental ability. "Who told you to do this?" asked the mercantilist.

"A girl. An ironsmith's daughter," the boy said.

"I was right," said the mercantilist, "but if you want to marry him off, let him get married to this smart girl."

"Wonderful," said the mother.

The mercantilist went to the hut where the girl lived with her parents, who were not home at the time. "They will be home soon," the girl said, letting the mercantilist into their humble home. "My dad has gone to buy a ruby for a cowrie, and mom has gone to market to sell words."

The mercantilist was perplexed, but he sat down to wait for the parents to return.

When the parents came back, they were shocked to see the rich mercantilist in their humble home, and they were more shocked when they heard that the mercantilist's son wanted to marry their daughter. Gossip about all this ran throughout the village, and some people began playing tricks by telling the stupid son that he should beat the ironsmith's daughter seven times a day to make her behave. (They thought that if the girl's father found out he would end this marriage). The stupid boy actually went to the girl's father and said he wanted to beat his future wife. The ironsmith wanted to end the marriage, but the girl did not. The night of the wedding, the stupid boy wanted to beat the girl with his shoe, but she said no, to wait, and if he wanted to beat her a week later, that was ok. But it was bad luck for a couple to fight their first week together.

The mercantilist's wife decided their now married son should have money to travel and invest. "No," the mercantilist said. "That's like throwing money in the river." But his wife talked him into it anyway.

The boy went out, traveling with a great caravan. He found a mansion in the midst of a garden where a most gorgeous woman coaxed him in for a game of chance. The stupid boy gambled away all of his money, losing it to this woman, including his servants and goods. When he was destitute, he was thrown into jail.

A man passing by the prison saw the young man and knew he came from his own country.

"Will you help me?" the boy called out to the man. "I can't pay my debts," said the stupid boy, and I must get these letters out to receive help from my father.

There were two letters—one he had written to his father, telling of his foolish deeds, and one to his wife, in which he lied and said he was successful and richer than ever before and would soon be home and beat her with his shoe.

The man who was to deliver the letters was illiterate, and he took the letters to the wrong people—the wife's to the father, and the father's to the wife. The father was happy about all the good fortune but didn't know why his son was saying he wanted to beat his father with a shoe when he got back. The wife wondered why he wrote to her about his troubles when his father had the money to bail him out. The father and daughter met, and it was decided that the wife would take money to get the boy out of jail. So the wife dressed up like a man and arrived at the palace, saying she was the son of a wealthy mercantilist. Of course, she was invited to gambol.

A game was started, and the wife was very wise and won back all her stupid husband had lost, as well as everything that the wicked gambling woman owned. The wife stayed in disguise, went to the prison and released all the prisoners. She now had the wicked woman and all her servants indebted to her and captive, and the whole entourage marched back to the mercantilist's and told him everything, while the stupid son went to his own house with all the money in boxes, except for one little box, which contained the stupid boy's dirty clothes from prison.

Later on, the stupid son went to see his parents and saw his wife was there. He began to take off one of his shoes to beat his wife.

"No!" said his parents, "What is the matter with you?"

His wife opened the box of his dirty clothes from prison and said, "Don't you remember wearing these?" She then revealed to him what she had done, pretending to be a man.

The boy's jaw dropped to the floor. The mercantilist and his wife were ashamed of their son and enamored of their daughter-in-law. "She is too good for him," said the mercantilist, and the wife finally agreed. "She keeps all the jewels and servants for herself," he proclaimed.[10]

14

LITERARY FILTERS

The more pity, that fools may not speak wisely what wise men do foolishly.

—William Shakespeare

All critical interpretations of literature raise specific filters through which stories, poems, and songs are perceived. In relationship to trickster stories, it is important to keep in mind that these tales are often from preliterate oral traditions (and translated into English from oral accounts) and would traditionally have ranked as belonging to "low" culture (even though most in academia would reject that assessment now). The stories often deal with base bodily functions and overt sexual acts. Like most myths, they don't make logical sense, even though there may be a "Why" story included (such as why bear lost his tail, or why men have a penis). In myths, the usual rules of daily life don't have to be followed—the dead don't have to stay dead for example. The following critical perspectives have both determined what texts were allowed into the literary canon (and taught at universities), and these theories have also created a historical body of meaning for texts. For this reason, I want to touch on some important critical positions over the last century that have had a large role in defining the nature and meaning of literature, and the validity of trickster tales as art worthy or not of critical commentary.

New Criticism (coming before Structuralism, arising in the 1920s and prominent through the 1960s) was itself a reaction against previous literary criticism that was seen as too subjective and lacking intellectual vigor. In trying to capture a more systematic method for evaluating literary works (once again, we see the constant *attempt* to ground literary studies in science), the founders of New Criticism developed what they saw as unbiased criteria from which to assess literature. Literature was to be examined through a "close reading" of the text alone, with everything outside the text, such as biography, history, culture deemed irrelevant. Attention to technique, and unity of effect, was called for, which was allegorically revealed in the title of Cleanth Brooks's treatise *The Well-Wrought Urn*. Literary art was to be constructed in the same way as a well-wrought urn should be—with symmetry, oppositional tensions, and aesthetic balance—and judged according to these properties. (No attention need be paid to who made the urn or for what purpose it was to be used.) New Criticism was a kind of formalism, in that the main critique and aesthetic concern had to do with formal properties. But in terms of analyzing trickster tales, New Criticism doesn't work. For the most part, these stories were told in cultures in which there was no word or concept for art. Authorship is usually not part of the mindset of storytellers, and there is nothing wrong when multiple versions of stories exist between storytellers who live right next to each other. The tales were not crafted with the design elements of New Criticism in mind and do not often follow such things as symmetry of design or balance that New Criticism saw as essential to art.

New Criticism focuses upon each art object but was replaced overall by Structuralism, which focuses upon larger categories. Structuralism itself was replaced by Post-Structuralism and Deconstruction, terms that stand for a loosely aligned set of theories that saw Structuralism as supporting power elites. The French theorists Derrida, Lacon, Barthes, and Foucalut argued that language itself evaded "all systems and logics" with a "'continual flickering, spilling and defusing of meaning,'" called by Derrida, "'dissemination'—which cannot be easily contained with categories to the text's structure, or within the categories of a conventional critical approach to it."[1] Ronald Barthes believed that any suggestion that language signs were natural was a sham, authoritarian, and ideological. The trickster figure, because of his distaste of power and his flexible nature, became a popular character for those in these camps. New Criticism held firm that there were empirical differences between high and low culture—Art/art, as did Frye within Structuralism (academia was always supposed to be concerned with high culture, as it was the role of the studied critic to interpret the literary "jewels"). But from the viewpoint of Deconstruction, language itself was seen as arbitrary, and the assertions of New Critics and Structuralists seemed completely indefensible. Trickster was a product of "low" culture, yet that did not mean he was not intriguing, entertaining, or an artistic creation. Postmodernist thinking revealed that the techniques of any critical approach could be applied to *any* work of art *or to any artifact of culture*, and any slotting of high or low was always a biased political act of categorization. This allowed for a reinterpretation of what "literature" is, for if the designation of literary itself was a political stance based on class and power; there was certainly no scientific validity to the process of privileging some texts over others. This led to a great opening up, for now the "literary canon" could no longer be justified in excluding texts of women, minorities, and oral cultures, for anything from a trickster tale from an illiterate tribe to a shopping list could be examined through creative acts of interpretation. This revelation had a profound (and I would say positive) affect on the academy, even though the overall affect of Deconstruction turned out to be an insane rejection of science.

The other dominant critical theory in the study of literature, since the 1970s, has been feminist theory, of which numerous branches have developed. Overall, feminist theory, arising during the same time period as Post-Structuralism, initially rejected the deconstructive approach of the French theorists, for Deconstruction did not include the "body," did not account for the *experience* of interacting with texts—emotion and feeling. The feminist movement showed that the perspective of women, their voices, their stories, literary production, and interpretation of literature, had been largely eliminated from the male-dominated academy and canon, and feminist theory rightfully set about to change that. Not only were many female literary voices resurrected, there was also a reinterpretation of *all* texts, male and female, from feminist perspectives. Feminism brought to light prejudice as well as the horrific and dominate patterns of male violence against women in societies around the world, which put feminism in conflict with male-dominated fundamentalist traditions worldwide. It was against broad misogynistic thinking that various streams of feminist literary criticism were born, and these eventually fractured into various "schools," a few different strains of which follow:

Liberal feminism, starting in the eighteenth century, takes the stance that "no special privileges for women [should be given] and demand[s] that everyone receive equal consideration without discrimination on the basis of sex."[2] Socialist feminism, is in stark contrast to liberal feminism, and sees "all knowledge as socially constructed and emerging from practical human involvement in production that takes a definite historic form."[3] African-American feminism comes from the position that race is the greatest oppressor, and rejects the individualism of liberal feminism as well as the Marxist assumption that class is at the heart of power struggles.[4] Socialist feminism is in stark contrast to liberal feminism, and sees "all knowledge as socially constructed and emerging from practical human involvement in production that takes a definite historic form."[5] Essentialist feminism takes the position that men and women are biologically different (based upon Darwinism). In the late 1800s, followers of this branch believed women to be inferior to men in some respects but superior in others. Contemporary followers of essentialist feminism have altered this to the belief that "biologically based differences between the sexes might imply superiority and power for women in some arenas."[6] Many feminist critics, however, have rejected Darwinian theory, including evolutionary psychology and biology, as it applies to differences between genders, for they see science itself as upholding traditional male prejudices against women. Some have joined in the Deconstructive belief that science itself is just another myth. As the work in cognitive science and evolutionary biology and psychology has become more dominant, this is changing in some quarters. Essentialist feminism, with its belief in the female mind being different than the male, has led to reinterpretations of the way science is conducted, while still believing overall in science. For instance, from this perspective such a question as this can be asked: Would Jane Goodall's ground-breaking, patient work with chimpanzees, taking place over decades, have ever been initiated by a man? Or are some kinds of research, approaches, even questions themselves, different when originating in the minds of women and men? Essentialists would answer yes. (Matt Ridley, in *The Red Queen*, objects, saying that "there is a contradiction at the heart of most feminism—or, one that few feminists have acknowledged. You cannot say, first, that men and women are equally capable of all jobs, and second, that if jobs were done by women, they would be done differently."[7])Radical feminism also sees most forms of knowledge as male-based, and therefore suspect.

Queer Studies came about from various other branches of feminist critique uniting, giving a positive voice to homosexuality, both male and female, as well as to all forms of sexual preference, taking a libertine stance, while also taking on the study of cultural reactions to sexuality. Queer studies, and its feminist links, have been one of the few feminist factions to embrace evolution and cognitive science, as science has continually shown that sexual preference is, in most cases, unlikely to be a matter of choice, but of biology—taking the stain of religious-based "sin" away from non-monogamous and homosexual acts.

As we have seen, Tricksters and Trickstars can be viewed in numerous ways, depending upon the theoretical lens from which one observes them. That Trickster often changes sex could be seen as inclusive to those in Queer studies, allowing androgyny, homosexuality, and transgenderism openly into narrative. But other feminists see Trickster as an abomination, another oppressive expression of male dominance. To Essentialists, a Darwinian view is accepted; to many Feminists, however, the Darwinian view contradicts social constructionist theory, that it is culture that shapes our lives, not genes, and feminism was founded upon 1960s ideals that males and females were different only because of society's instruction, not genes.

Cultural Studies and Semiotics (where much Trickster scholarship resides), are critical areas that combine elements of Post-Modernism, Post-Structuralism, and Deconstruction, with the focus usually being upon the question of how texts exist within larger cultural concepts of ideology, nationality, ethnicity, and the distribution of power. In semiotics, the interpretation of symbols, or signs, allows the researcher to mine below the surface of imagery and assess unconscious psychological motives and cultural signifiers not readily apparent on the surface (interestingly enough, also a Structuralist goal).

Cognitive Narrative Theory (as my own inquiry entails) takes scientific gleanings from neuroscience and biology on how the brain works to examine language, texts, and story structure. Literature is examined for insights into the cognitive and evolutionary processes they might reveal.

There are others modes of literary interpretation of course, but the study of Trickster has been impacted in numerous ways by all of the theoretical positions discussed. Trickster was interpreted as a Jungian "archetype"; seen as evidence of Structuralist validity; embraced by Post-Structrualism and Deconstruction for his liminal quality (the fact that he can shape-shift and change form, inhabiting numerous environments with multiple meanings, simultaneously, in the same way that language is seen to be constantly in flux without core meaning). Trickster has been seen in some feminist camps as representing the nightmare of male excess and penetration, while other feminists see the male trickster as a kind of cautionary tale, warning females of men's motives and desires, while the Trickstar, the female version of Trickster, has been perceived as a champion who often prevails through greater wit and intelligence, through subverting the world of men. Cultural Studies scholars often use the trickster archetype to explain the existence of comedic and rebellious characters from *I Love Lucy* to *The Simpsons* to *Wile E. Coyote*. Semiotics writers revel in Trickster as signifying multiple perspectives that are dynamic and in constant flux, while Deconstructionists (and Marxists) will also see in Trickster a political force who is continually challenging the status quo, turning the tables on the rich and powerful, on hierarchy itself. For a Cognitive Narrative Analysis, the workings of the brain are sought after through examining ways in which language and stories are created and transferred to the community: Trickster is seen here as a manifestation that allows us a glimpse into both our current and ancient selves rooted in the biological process of evolution.

⑮

MUSIC AND THE TRICKSTER

Without music life would be a mistake.

—Nietzsche

If music be the food of love, play on.

—Williams Shakespeare

It is no accident that one of the first tasks the Old Testament God gives to Adam is that of naming the animals. Language categorizes our world, divides it into nouns, subjects, and objects; and it mimics the animation of moving, living things through verbs. Such power is part of the trickster's realm, the "silver-tongued-devil" who can manipulate rhetoric to his own advantage, akin to the ancient Greek Sophists, who Plato despised for their ability to speak from both sides of their mouth, artfully. For the Fon of Africa, Legba, the trickster figure, is also known as the "divine linguist" who

> speaks all languages, he who interprets the alphabet of Mawu to man and to the other gods. Yoruba sculptures of Esu almost always include a calabash that he holds in his hands. In this calabash he keeps *ase*, the very *ase* with which Olodumare, the supreme deity of the Yoruba, created the

universe. We can translate *ase* in many words, but the *ase* used to create
the universe I translate as 'logos,' as the word as understanding, the word
as audible, and later the visible, ordinary word. It is the word with irrevo-
cability, reinforced with double assuredness and undaunted authenticity.
This probably explains why Esu's mouth, from which the audible word
proceeds, sometimes appears double; Esu's discourse, metaphorically,
is double-voiced. Esu's mastery of *ase* gives him an immense amount of
power; *ase* makes Esu "he who says so and does so."[1]

Likewise, the beginning of the world in the Old Testament initiates
from the voice of God: "And God said, let there be light and there was
light." In the New Testament, Jesus is also identified with the logos in
John: "In the beginning was the Word, and the Word was with God,
and the Word was God." Language is power, and in ancient times words
were thought to have magical properties. But the greatest power of all
regarding language has always been in the form of song.

When God blows his breath into Adam's nostrils, it is akin to a song,
Adam becoming the musical instrument of God. Moses—a kind of trickster himself for all his magical abilities—surviving as a baby in a reed
ark, talking with a burning bush, holding a magic staff (like Hermes),
sending plagues, causing God to open the sea, going up to the mountain-
top for visions for the inscribed words of God, having God drop manna
from heaven, is himself associated with song:

> Then sang Moses and the children of Israel this song unto the LORD, and
> spake, saying, I will sing unto the LORD, for he hath triumphed glori-
> ously: the horse and his rider hath he thrown into the sea. The LORD is
> my strength and song, and he is become my salvation: he is my God, and
> I will prepare him an habitation; my father's God, and I will exalt him.
>
> Moses therefore wrote this song the same day, and taught it the chil-
> dren of Israel.[4] And Moses spake in the ears of all the congregation of
> Israel the words of this song, until they were ended. And Moses came and
> spake all the words of this song in the ears of the people, he, and Hoshea
> the son of Nun.

In the African story, "Iyadola's Babies," "two spirit people [are]
sneezed out of the mouth of the Creator." There are countless creation stories where breath, wind, voice, initiate the magic of life. And

for ancient, preliterate, and primal people, song—breath and voice at its greatest pitch—was the mainstay of literature. Songs were used for everything—to rock a child to sleep, to still the wind, to bring the rain, to heal the sick, to prepare for war, to put parents to sleep so that a man might enter the tepee of his beloved, or to bury the dead. Even in our own culture, we use songs to consecrate our most significant and ceremonial events—a baptism, a graduation, a catechism or bar mitzvah, a seduction of a lover, a birthday, a funeral. Music—with the inclusion of rhythm—is no doubt the oldest of the arts, stemming from the very movement of our bodies, the beating of our hearts, and it seems to have a mysterious force that works on us in ways nothing else does. As we have seen with chimpanzees, there may be a glimpse of the first song in their rain dances. And of course many animals sing—everything from the howling of wolves to the multitude of bird songs throughout the world. It was Darwin who first brought up the idea that human song must have had its origins in our proto-human phase of existence for reasons similar to the development of song in other species.

For primal people, songs are a way of keeping the mind, body and the natural world in order. Poems, as we have seen, in preliterate societies, are always songs. And prayer is usually song as well. A. LaVonne Brown Ruoff, writing of harmony in American Indian traditional culture between the psychic and physical universe states that

> balance [is] vital to an individual and communal sense of wholeness or beauty . . . [and that] breath, speech, and verbal art are so closely linked to each other that in many oral cultures they are often signified by the same word. The reverence for the power of thought and the word that is an integral part of American Indian religions is exemplified in Navajo culture. In *Language and Art in the Navajo Universe*, Gary Witherspoon points out that the Navajo world was brought into being by the gods, who entered the sweathouse and thought the world into existence. The thoughts of the gods were realized through human speech, song, and prayer.[2]

In times of great emotion nothing else will do but song. Nearly all healing through shamanistic rituals is accompanied by song. Songs are often the primary way tribal people communicate with their deities. Songs in trickster tales are often present—during acts of creation, during sexual seduction, during healing, and in a host of other moments in which song breaks forth to punctuate life. In many trickster stories, such as the Yoruba tales from West Africa, Trickster is well known as a musician, and music is an integral part of his rapscallion personality as well as his method of seduction. This brings us back to the Ornamental Mind theory of Miller and the Courting Arts Darwin saw as the antecedent to music, poetry, and song. Evolutionary theory predicts that we should see a link between the arts, sexual selection, seduction, and procreation, which we continually do.

The following origin stories give an insight into the primacy of music in the origin myths of various primal people in which the Creator instigates the big bang with the help of song. In some there appear obvious combinations of Christian and aboriginal elements.

SINGING THE WORLD INTO BEING: CREATION STORIES WITH SONG

Apache Creation Story (North America)

In the beginning nothing existed—no earth, no sky, no sun, no moon, only darkness was everywhere.

Suddenly from the darkness emerged a thin disc, one side yellow and the other side white, appearing suspended in midair. Within the disc sat a small bearded man, Creator, the One Who Lives Above. As if waking from a long nap, he rubbed his eyes and face with both hands.

When he looked into the endless darkness, light appeared above. He looked down and it became a sea of light. To the east, he created yellow streaks of dawn. To the west, tints of many colours appeared everywhere. There were also clouds of different colors.

Creator wiped his sweating face and rubbed his hands together, thrusting them downward. Behold! A shining cloud upon which sat a little girl.

"Stand up and tell me where are you going," said Creator. But she did not reply. He rubbed his eyes again and offered his right hand to the Girl-Without-Parents.

"Where did you come from?" she asked, grasping his hand.

"From the east where it is now light," he replied, stepping upon her cloud.

"Where is the earth?" she asked.

"Where is the sky?" he asked, and sang, "I am thinking, thinking, thinking what I shall create next." He sang four times, which was the magic number.

Creator brushed his face with his hands, rubbed them together, then flung them wide open! Before them stood Sun-God. Again Creator rubbed his sweaty brow and from his hands dropped Small-Boy.

All four gods sat in deep thought upon the small cloud.

"What shall we make next?" asked Creator. "This cloud is much too small for us to live upon."

Then he created Tarantula, Big Dipper, Wind, Lightning-Maker, and some western clouds in which to house Lightning-Rumbler, which he just finished.

Creator sang, "Let us make earth. I am thinking of the earth, earth, earth; I am thinking of the earth," he sang four times.

All four gods shook hands. In doing so, their sweat mixed together and Creator rubbed his palms, from which fell a small round, brown ball, not much larger than a bean.

Creator kicked it, and it expanded. Girl-Without-Parents kicked the ball, and it enlarged more. Sun-God and Small-Boy took turns giving it hard kicks, and each time the ball expanded. Creator told Wind to go inside the ball and to blow it up.

Tarantula spun a black cord and, attaching it to the ball, crawled away fast to the east, pulling on the cord with all his strength. Tarantula repeated with a blue cord to the south, a yellow cord to the west, and a white cord to the north. With mighty pulls in each direction, the brown ball stretched to immeasurable size—it became the earth! No hills, mountains, or rivers were visible; only smooth, treeless, brown plains appeared.

Creator scratched his chest and rubbed his fingers together and there appeared Hummingbird.

"Fly north, south, east, and west and tell us what you see," said Creator.

"All is well," reported Hummingbird upon his return. "The earth is most beautiful, with water on the west side."

But the earth kept rolling and dancing up and down. So Creator made four giant posts—black, blue, yellow, and white to support the earth. Wind carried the four posts, placing them beneath the four cardinal points of the earth. The earth sat still.

Creator sang, "World is now made and now sits still," which he repeated four times.[3]

Bunjil the Creator, No. 1 (Aboriginal, Australian)

Bunjil was not satisfied until he had created sentient human beings. It was a harder task than any he had attempted. The making of other forms of animal life had been comparatively simple. The marking of a man was a challenge to the Great Spirit, for within the framework of flesh there was need for powers of thought, reasoning, and other human characteristics that would separate man from the animal creation.

He pondered long before attempting the supreme masterpiece. When at last he was ready he prepared two sheets of bark, cutting them to the shape he envisaged as suited to such a noble purpose. Mobility and dexterity were important, and these he incorporated into his design. Next he took soft clay, molding it to the shape of the bark, smoothing it with his hands.

When the work was finished he danced round the two inert figures, implanting seeds of knowledge and the capacity to reason and learn.

The time had come for his skill to be put to the test. He gave them names—Berrook-boorn and Kookin-berrook. This was the first and most important step, for without names they would have lacked personality and spirit. Bunjil was well aware that if these beings were to fulfill their purpose, they must share his spirit as well as the characteristics of animals.

Although without breath, they were now named and ready for the infilling of the life force. Again Bunjil danced round them and then lay on their bodies, one after the other, breathing breath and life into their mouths, nostrils, and navels.

For the third time Bunjil danced round them. As his feet wove intricate patterns in the dust, Berrook-boorn and Kookin-berrook rose slowly to their feet. They linked hands with Bunjil and with each other, joining the All-Father in the dance of life, singing with him the first song that ever came from the lips of man.[4]

Diné (or Navajo) (North America)

According to the Diné, they emerged from three previous underworlds into this, the fourth, or "Glittering World," through a magic reed. The first people from the other three worlds were not like the people of today. They were animals, insects, or masked spirits as depicted in Navajo ceremonies. First Man ('Altsé Hastiin), and First Woman ('Altsé 'Asdzáá), were two of the beings from the First or Black World. First Man was made in the east from the meeting of the white and black clouds. First Woman was made in the west from the joining of the yellow and blue clouds. Spider Woman (Na ashje'ii 'Asdzáá), who taught Navajo women how to weave, was also from the first world.

Once in the Glittering World, the first thing the people did was build a sweat house and sing the Blessing Song.[5]

MYTHIC TRICKSTER MUSICIANS AND SINGERS

As we have seen, music and language in all probability stem from the same root, music being older, with both emerging primarily due to sexual selection as courtship strategies, and the link between sexuality and music is absolutely clear in many trickster stories. In his introduction to *Yoruba Trickster Tales*, Oyekan Owomoyela gives a succinct description of the character of Ajapa, the Trickster who appears as Tortoise, one of his chief characteristics being his musical genius.

No discussion of Ajapa can ignore one of his most remarkable accomplishments: his irresistible musicianship. In many tales his scheme is carried by his singing, which casts a powerful spell on individuals and whole communities, even on other-wordly beings, so that they forget themselves and their present purpose, abandoning themselves to the rhythm of his songs.

But perhaps the Trickster's most impressive endowments are his inde-
structibility and immortality, qualities that might justify those instances in
which he is elevated to the status of a god.

Ajapa and the Roasted Peanut Seller (Yoruba, Africa)

*There once lived in Ajapa's town a woman famous for the incredible,
mouth-watering roasted peanuts she prepared and sold at the daily market. Each day market people waited expectantly for the breeze to waft
the aroma of roasting peanuts to their nostrils, signaling them either
to make their way to the woman's stall or to send a child or servant to
purchase some of the treat. They simply would not feel right about starting their day until they had satisfied the craving the irresistible aroma
unfailingly provoked in them.*

*There was no more faithful market-goer than Ajapa, not because he had
anything to sell, for he was incurably lazy and incapable of addressing
himself to any productive venture, not because he had anything to buy, for
without producing anything he lacked the means to purchase anything.
No, he was religiously at the market each day because he could always
find some compassionate trader to extend some alms to him. Yet each day
at the market was also torture to him, because like everybody else, his gul-
let involuntarily commenced to swallow emptiness whenever the smell of
roasted peanuts reached his nose. Unfortunately, that was one commodity
no one seemed willing to share with him, and the peanut seller was herself
a hard-hearted woman as far as Ajapa was concerned. Nothing he did, no
plea he made softened her to offer him even a taste of her peanuts.*

*"You made no gash in the palm-tree, nor did you sling a shot to pierce
the pate of the wine-producing tree, yet go to its base and expectantly
uplift your open mouth. Do you think pal-wine flows of its own accord?"
she sneered at him in response to his importunity.*

*The scolding was salt on Ajapa's wounded pride, and being who he
was, it was not long before his frustration and anger triggered his propensity for mischief, and he set about devising a way to get his fill of the
delicious peanuts despite the mean seller. He sought out Okere the Giant Rat, who was renowned for his great burrowing prowess, and asked
what it would take to get him to dig a tunnel from the nearby forest to
the peanut woman's stall in the market. Okete assured Ajapa that if the*

latter would provide him with a sackful of peanuts he could consider the job as good as done. For once Ajapa submitted himself to the necessity of self-exertion; he scoured the bases of tens of palm-trees in the forests around, gathering the nuts scattered thereabouts, and before long he had the sackful to pay Okete. The latter lost no time in setting to work as he promised, and in no more than two days the tunnel was ready, its mouth right by the peanut seller's seat. Under cover of night Ajapa sneaked into the market and concealed the opening with dried leaves so expertly that no one could suspect its presence. That done, he went home to await the propitious time when, as he told himself, the boil that had long plagued him would at last be lanced.

At daybreak, market-goers flocked to their stalls as usual, and so did the peanut seller. The day had dawned like any other, offering no hint that it harbored any surprise for the traders, but Ajapa had installed himself at the mouth of the tunnel just below the leaf covering, armed with his drum and ready to act as soon as his nostrils announced to him the moment. He could not see any of the above-ground activity from his concealment, but he could hear it all. From there his keen nose registered the progress of the peanut roasting, and when he was satisfied that the seller had roasted a sufficiently large amount, he applied the stick to his drum and launched into song:

> *Peanut seller, do lend an ear,*
> *Crackle, crackle, pop!*
> *Peanut seller, please hear my song,*
> *Crackle, crackle, pop!*
> *Shouldn't you be dancing?*
> *Crackle, crackle, pop!*
> *Yield yourself to my music,*
> *Crackle, crackle, pop!*
> *Leave your stall in my care,*
> *Crackle, crackle, pop!*
> *You really should be dancing!*
> *Crackle, crackle, pop!*
> *Peanuts, crackling and popping,*
> *Crackle, crackle, pop!*
> *Peanuts, crackling,* and *popping,*
> *Crackle, crackle, pop!*

Had Ajapa but known it, and had he not been perversely addicted to idleness, he would have acknowledged his true calling and lived gainfully by it. For in truth few creatures were capable of making music as irresistible as his, music that could set the most reluctant feet dancing with abandon in spite of themselves. The effect of his performance on the peanut seller, on her customers, and indeed on everybody in the market was as Ajapa hoped. All gave way to dance with such vigor that they were soon enveloped in a cloud of dust, and in the time it would take a crab to blink their momentum had carried them almost to the other end of town. It did not matter that the music that got them dancing had long stopped, and they had danced so far from its source anyway that they could not have heard it even if it had not. Befuddled and shamefaced, they returned like suddenly sober drunkards to the market, where they found the peanut seller's roasted nuts completely gone. No other stall had been disturbed.

She raised the alarm, and people quickly established a connection between the new musical phenomenon that had intruded into their midst and the disappearance of the peanuts. They had no option in such circumstances but to report the incident to the oba, in whose charge the welfare of the town lay.

Since the market was close to his palace, occupying a large open expanse in front of it, in fact, the oba had himself been aware of the unusual commotion, and he was therefore not entirely surprised when his people trooped into his courtyard and asked for an urgent audience. On hearing the peanut seller's story he concluded that the culprit must be a clever rascal, a daytime rogue with a taste for roasted peanuts. He consulted with his chiefs, who advised him to assign the task of apprehending the culprit and preventing a repetition of the visitation to the seasoned hunters of the town, whose task was also to keep thieves and burglars at bay.

Dutifully, then, all the hunters gathered on the market day following, sporting their fearful weapons and festooned with powerful amulets and charms. However intrepid the rascal, he was about to discover the mettle of the town's hunters, they vowed. A huge crowd, much larger than usually found at the market, had gathered to witness the confrontation between hunters and peanut fiend. The hunters kept the crowd back as best they could, positioned themselves around the peanut stall, and asked the seller to commence her usual activities. She obliged and began to roast peanuts, but for a while nothing happened. Then, after she had roasted a sizable heap of nuts, and just as the hunters and some in the crowd were becoming convinced that the phantom singer had allowed good sense to master his wayward appetite, the singing began:

> Peanut seller, do lend an ear,
> Crackle, crackle, pop!
> Peanut seller, please hear my song,
> Crackle, crackle, pop!
> Shouldn't you be dancing?
> Crackle, crackle, pop!
> Yield yourself to my music,
> Crackle, crackle, pop!
> Leave your stall in my care,
> Crackle, crackle, pop!
> You really should be dancing!
> Crackle, crackle, pop!
> Peanuts, crackling and popping,
> Crackle, crackle, pop!
> Peanuts, crackling and popping,
> Crackle, crackle, pop!

When some time later the hunters came to their senses and found themselves amidst the market crowd, bereft of their weapons, medicines, and charms, they knew something had gone badly awry. On looking around and recognizing their whereabouts, the end of town farthest from the market, they could not look one another in the face. This time the townspeople had no need to be embarrassed: rather they directed their mirthful ridicule at the hunters, making snide remarks about weapons that were no better than dancing staffs. The whole crowd trooped back to the market to find what they knew they would find: a depleted stock of peanuts.

The hunter's disgrace convinced the oba of the severity of the problem on his hands. If his hunters were powerless against the mysterious thief, perhaps he was no mere human after all; perhaps the creature was an iwin, a fairy. With that suspicion in mind he sought the intervention of his diviners and medicine men. They gathered at the market on the next market day bristling with their own charms and assorted paraphernalia,

*all ready to make an end of whatever it was that plagued their town or
at least teach it to give it a wide berth thenceforward. When the singing began, however, not even these masters of mysteries could control
themselves. They surrendered to the music just as all the others had done
before them.*

*Once sober again, the town was thrown into a panic, for even though
the mysterious musical creature seemed interested only in peanuts, it
nevertheless kept everyone from their trading. Moreover, any phenomenon that could humble the trusted hunters and medicine men could also
wreak greater havoc on the town if it chose. It had to be stopped. The
oba could think of nowhere else to turn but to the Osanyin clan. These
were humanlike spirits endowed with great magical powers, and they
regularly held commerce with humans as trouble-solvers of last resort,
especially when the trouble involved other spirits. In appearance they
were very much like humans, differing only with regard to how many
legs they had: whereas humans normally had two, an Osanyin could
have as many as ten legs and as few as one, but they could not have
two, for a two-legged Osanyin would hardly be distinguishable from a
human. When the oba turned to them for help, the ten-legged patriarch
Osanyin assured him that he and his town would be rid of the music-
playing, peanut-stealing wonder the next day. He gave instructions for
the peanut seller and other marketers to carry out their routine the following day and leave matters to him.*

*The patriarch assigned the task first to the three-legged Osanyin, the
one-legged one being considered so handicapped that the idea of his confronting the phenomenon was thought ludicrous. The next morning the
first creature at the market was the prospective hero of the day, the three-
legged Osanyin. Before anyone else arrived he pronounced fearsome incantations on the peanut seller's stall and its vicinity, incantations designed to
confuse and paralyze any wayward spirit that might venture near there.
In time the market filled up, this time with the oba and his councilors in
attendance. They would not miss the confrontation of spirits, nor a sight
of the thing that had so disrupted the life of the town these past few days.*

*When all was ready, the Osanyin gave the word, and the peanut seller
began roasting her peanuts. For a while nothing happened, until she
had filled her calabash with a sizable mound of roasted peanuts, and the
aroma suffused the air of the whole town. Then the music commenced:*

Peanut seller, do lend an ear,
Crackle, crackle, pop!
Peanut seller, please hear my song,
Crackle, crackle, pop!
Shouldn't you be dancing?
Crackle, crackle, pop!
Yield yourself to my music,
Crackle, crackle, pop!
Leave your stall in my care,
Crackle, crackle, pop!
You really should be dancing!
Crackle, crackle, pop!
Peanuts, crackling and popping,
Crackle, crackle, pop!
Peanuts, crackling and popping,
Crackle, crackle, pop!

The Osanyin danced so hard that he danced two of his legs off, and the oba and his councilors were indistinguishable from the ordinary people when the effects of the music wore off and they found themselves well away from the market.

Unable to bear the disgrace, the Osanyin clan went into conclave and vowed to bring the musical spirit to hell or permanently remove themselves from the vicinity of the town. They sent the four-legged Osanyin into the fray, but he also proved a failure; he lost three legs! The same fate befell the five-legged Osanyin and then the six-legged. To make a long story short, all the others, including the most powerful of them all, the ten-legged patriarch Osanyin, failed in their confrontation with the musical phenomenon, and they prepared to remove themselves into disgraceful exile.

Now the oba himself was in a panic. The chief duty the ancestors entrusted to him was to keep the town and the community secure, and on his departure from this life to hand them in full security to his successor. If in his time the town was laid waste because some unknown creature disrupted its life, what report would he give to those who preceded him when he was reunited with them in the afterlife? But just when he felt most hopeless, the oba found the one-legged Osanyin standing before him.

"The crown will live long on your head, your Majesty," he greeted the oba.

"So be it," the latter responded rather listlessly.

"The shoes will stay long on your feet," the Osanyin continued.

"So be it," the oba responded again, almost showing his impatience at this visit from one of the failed clan of Osanyin. He had too much on his mind for pleasantries.

"You have a message for me, perhaps, from the rest of your kin?" he asked.

"No, your Majesty," the visitor responded. "I came on my own."

"Well. . . ?"

"It is about the nuisance that's causing you and your town all this trouble."

"Yes?" the oba said questioningly.

"I will catch and deliver him to you," the Osanyin said matter-of-factly.

"You?" the oba asked, hardly able to keep the incredulity from his voice.

There was a glint in his eyes, but one of wonderment. The creature was serious, but he was also being ridiculous, the oba thought. As the saying went, if an ago, the smartest of rats, fell victim to the snare, what chance had the olose, the most sluggish of rodents?

"I know what you are thinking, your Majesty," his visitor said. "The Osanyin who had more limbs than I failed at the task, so how can I accomplish it? Remember, though, the needle may be tiny, but it is nothing for a chick to swallow. Let me at the troublesome wretch. If I succeed, you are well rid of the nuisance. If I fail, you would hardly be any worse off than you are now."

The oba considered the offer and consulted with the chiefs sitting around him. In the end he agreed with his visitor. Since the town stood to lose nothing from the Esenin's try, he might as well be given an opportunity to prove himself. He needed three days to prepare, he said, after which he would be at the market to take on the musical nuisance.

When the appointed day arrived, the market was so crowded that there was no room for one more foot or one more arm. In the crowd were the Osanyin whose earlier efforts had failed, very angry and present only in anticipation of the pleasure of laughing at their overreaching, upstart *kin. The one-legged* Osanyin *had come armed with a sharp iron spike and nothing else—nothing, that is, except the cotton he had stuffed into his ears. He stuck his iron spike into the peanut seller's fire until its tip glowed white-hot. Then he instructed the woman to commence roasting peanuts. Soon there was a small mountain of roasted peanuts in the calabash, and as the crowd had expected, the music started:*

> *Peanut seller, do lend an ear,*
> *Crackle, crackle, pop!*
> *Peanut seller, please hear my song,*
> *Crackle, crackle, pop!*
> *Shouldn't you be dancing?*
> *Crackle, crackle, pop!*
> *Yield yourself to my music,*
> *Crackle, crackle, pop!*
> *Leave your stall in my care,*
> *Crackle, crackle, pop!*
> *You really should be dancing!*
> *Crackle, crackle, pop!*
> *Peanuts, crackling and popping,*
> *Crackle, crackle, pop!*
> *Peanuts, crackling and popping,*
> *Crackle, crackle, pop!*

As usual, the whole assemblage succumbed to dancing, including even the other Osanyin *whose restored limbs had not quite healed. Very soon all that could be seen of the dancers was the cloud of dust that trailed them as their gyrating movements carried them farther and farther away. As for the one-legged* Osanyin, *having stuffed his ears with cotton he heard none of the music, and having one leg only, he would not have felt the urge to dance, anyway. He spared only one glance for the disappearing crowd before riveting his eyes again on the stall.*

Soon he noticed the ground moving under the peanut seller's abandoned seat. Carefully, he withdrew his iron spike from the fire and held it ready to strike. In a short while Ajapa had cleared the dry-leaf cover over the hole and was in plain sight. His eyes and mind were so fixed on the peanuts that he paid no attention to whatever or whoever else might be around as he closed in on them—until he felt a powerful, muscle-

jerking, burning, piercing sensation in his nose. He writhed in pain, but his adversary was unrelenting. The Osanyin's spike went all the way through Agapa's nose and impaled him to the ground. He screamed and squirmed painfully, but the Osanyin showed no mercy. Ajapa became weaker and weaker, until satisfied that there was little fight left in him, the Osanyin relieved his pressure, lifted him up, and carried him to the oba's palace.

There Ajapa was put on display for the returning crowd to see. No one would believe that Ajapa could have had such powers on them, but they had the testimony of their eyes, the words of the oba and the Osanyin, and the confession of the culprit himself. As for Ajapa's fate, the oba decreed that it was only fitting that he spend the rest of his life serving the agent who proved powerful enough to apprehend him.

Thus Ajapa became a servant to the Osanyin, and thus it came to be that to this day the sacrifice offered to an Osanyin is a tortoise. If anyone ever heard Ajapa's speech he or she would notice its pronounced nasality, the enduring legacy of the Osanyin's spike.[6]

Coyote Giving (Paiute, North America)

Every man should have his own song, and no one else should be allowed to sing it, unless the owner permits it. At the high points in a man's life, when he kills his first deer, when he first makes love to a woman, out of this kind of happening he makes up his own song. He sings his song on great occasions. He might leave it to his son.

There was a man called No-Song. They called him that because this poor man owned no song. At a corn dance or a rain dance he would sit apart from the others. Often he tried to hide or lose himself in a crowd, because people would point him out to each other, saying: "Over there is that pitiful man who has no song." And because of his sad condition, he was too shy to court the young maidens.

So one day this man No-Song had harvested a big load of corn. He also had a big pot bubbling full of delicious venison stew. Coyote smelled it from afar. Coyote came running. "Oh, my," he thought, "I must get this corn, I must get this wonderful stew!" He was slavering. He said: "Hey, No-Song, what will you swap for your corn and for that sweet-smelling stew?"

"You are Coyote, the Song-Maker. You can have all this for a song."

"What kind of song?" asked Coyote.

"A song that will make the heart of young women butter," said No-Song. "I wish for a song to make glad the people so that they will admire me. Also I don't want a Coyote song, because Coyotes are the kind of fellows who want to take their gifts back."

"I would never do something so bad," said Coyote, whose mouth kept on watering.

"Give me your word that this will not be what they call a 'Coyote giving.'"

"I promise, I promise, as long as the song is wisely used for its purpose—to court a maiden and, on a special occasion, to gladden the hearts of the people."

"How can you think that I would not use the song in the right way?" said No-Song, somewhat insulted. Then Coyote gave him a song and he gave to Coyote all the corn and the big pot of venison stew. Both were very happy with the bargain they had made.

Soon there was held a great feast and dance, a fine occasion for No-Song to sing. All the people were astonished and delighted at this song. "How come," they asked, "suddenly No-Song can sing so sweetly?"

All the people clapped their hands and expressed their delight. At once a beautiful maiden suggested to No-Song that they should go behind some bushes, to a hidden place, and there do something that the teller of this story will not elaborate upon. And No-Song went from feast to feast, and from dance to dance, singing his song, and all who heard it were enchanted. And No-Song changed his name to "Singing Wonderfully."

Now, this singing of his song had gone on for months, and he had sung his song wherever he found people to listen, and their praise went to his head. And the one who called himself Singing Wonderfully sang his song for many purposes for which it was not designed, and he sang it so often that people grew bored with it and fell asleep while he was singing. And so, one night when this man calling himself Singing Wonderfully was asleep, Coyote crept up to him and took the song back. Coyote felt justified in doing this, because Singing Wonderfully had misused the song. And when the singer awoke, the song was gone. He could not remember a single word of it and neither could anyone else.

And the people called him No-Song again. So now he is sitting there every day with a huge bag of corn before him and a huge bubbling pot of venison stew, but, so far, Coyote has not come back.[7]

Hermes (Greek)

Hermes, the herald of the Olympian gods, is the son of Zeus and the nymph Maia, daughter of Atlas and one of the Pleiades. Hermes is the god of shepherds, land travel, merchants, weights and measures, oratory, literature, athletics, and thieves, and known for his cunning and shrewdness. More importantly, he is the messenger of the gods. Besides that he was also a minor patron of poetry. He was worshipped throughout Greece—especially in Arcadia—and festivals in his honor were called Hermoea.

According to legend, Hermes was born in a cave on Mount Cyllene in Arcadia. Zeus had impregnated Maia in the dead of night while all other gods slept. When dawn broke amazingly he was born. Maia wrapped him in swaddling bands, then resting herself, fell fast asleep. Hermes, however, squirmed free and ran off to Thessaly. This is where Apollo, his brother, grazed his cattle. Hermes stole a number of the heard and drove them back to Greece. He hid them in a small grotto near to the city of Pylos and covered their tracks. Before returning to the cave he caught a tortoise, killed it, and removed its entrails. Using the intestines from a cow stolen from Apollo and the hollow tortoise shell, he made the first lyre. When he reached the cave he wrapped himself back into the swaddling bands. When Apollo realized he had been robbed he protested to Maia that it had been Hermes who had taken his cattle. Maia looked to Hermes and said it could not be, as he was still wrapped in swaddling bands. Zeus the all powerful intervened saying he had been watching and Hermes should return the cattle to Apollo. As the argument went on, Hermes began to play his lyre. The sweet music enchanted Apollo, and he offered Hermes to keep the cattle in exchange for the lyre. Apollo later became the grand master of the instrument, and it also became one of his symbols. Later while Hermes watched over his herd he invented the pipes known as syrinx (pan-pipes), which he made from reeds. Hermes was also credited with inventing the flute. Apollo, also desired this instrument, so Hermes bartered with Apollo and received his golden wand which Hermes later used as his heralds staff. (In other versions Zeus gave Hermes his heralds staff.)[8]

Hanuman (India)

In India, the god Hanuman, himself a manifestation of Shiva (the reincarnation of his eleventh incarnation, Rudra) is a trickster with the head and tail of a monkey and the body of a man. As soon as he was born he was unnaturally hungry:

> Looking all around in the forest for something to eat, he caught sight of the sun. Mistaking it for a red fruit, he leapt into the firmament and seized it to devour. The Sun got terrified and shrieked and shouted for help.[9]

One version of the story has the Sun hiding in Indra's heaven, with Indra hurling a thunderbolt at baby Hanuman, who is injured on the chin. After this Brahma gathers the gods and blesses Hanuman with great gifts of brilliance, oratory, health, wealth, and more. He goes back to the forest to be raised by his parents, becoming a prankster of a youth, cursed by muteness by irritated rishis trying to meditate, with the stipulation being that the curse could only be lifted when Hanuman was reminded of his gifts. Eventually his voice returns, and through education he develops even more superior skills—the ability to assume any shape or size and to become invisible; the power of great military genius; psychic powers; the ability to fly; great oratory, scholarship, and musical genius—even to the point where he creates a theory of music, for which the gods give him honor.[10]

South Indian sculptors appear to have been particularly fascinated by the artistic facets of Hanuman's personality. Temples all over this region, from Andhra Pradesh downwards, are embellished with reliefs featuring the god striking an elegant dancing pose or playing on musical instruments. The bronze icons portray him in the same postures, entranced by devotional songs and music, wielding berena, cymbals and a manuscript or simply singing praises of his beloved lord Shri Rama.[11]

Scholars are uncertain as to the origin of Hanuman, whether he was originally a pre-Vedic tribal deity or arose later. But the stories of Hanuman traveled throughout Asia, Buddhists monks carrying the stories

of Hanuman as they traveled, retelling the tales with various versions
(promoting the concept of the Bodhisattva, a Buddhist version of the
"saint" in Mahayana tradition, who gives up claim to entering nirvana
until all sentient beings can first be saved) which radiated from China
to Java to Japan, many of them becoming incorporated into the national
literature of various Asian countries. In Southeast Asian stories, Hanuman is considered a philanderer, contrary to the tradition of him being
celibate in Indian tradition, once again incorporating one of the most
salient of Trickster characteristics.

The Zande Trickster, Tule; The Bushman (Africa)

In the introduction to *The Zande Trickster*, E. E. Evans-Pritchard states
that Tule is a monster of depravity: liar, cheat, lecher, murderer; vain,
greedy, treacherous, ungrateful, a poltroon, a braggart. This utterly selfish person is everything against which Azande warn their children most
strongly. Yet he is the hero of their stories, and it is to their children
that his exploits are related and he is presented, with very little moral-
izing—if as a rogue, as an engaging one. For there is another side to his
character, which even to us is appealing: his whimsical fooling, reckless-
ness, impetuosity, puckish irresponsibility, his childish desire to show
how clever he is, his total absorption in song and dance, his feathered
hat, and his flouting of every convention.[12]

16

A SWATH OF OTHER TRICKSTER
STORIES FROM AROUND THE WORLD

If the fool would persist in his folly he would become wise.

—William Blake

As said before, what exactly makes a story a "trickster" story is hard to pin down, as there are so many manifestations of Trickster from culture to culture, and even within cultures there are often many varieties of the Trickster, representing the entire spectrum of good and evil, funny and serious, male and female. But there is almost always some "trick" in which change occurs and the status quo is interrupted (or at least an attempt is made for such). In the Monkey King we see the shape-shifting, foolish, and ego-driven monkey move from a kind of rogue to a cultural hero—even becoming a Buddha. In this he represents the move from a rascal toward an awakened mind, leaving behind what is often called in Buddhism the "monkey mind." From the point of view of neuroscience, this is a metaphor for saying that the neocortex finds a way of controlling the amygdala, the basal ganglia, and all rest of the more primitive parts of the brain, though the greater lesson of both Buddhism and neuroscience is that these "parts" of ourselves are not apart—they all make up who we are—there is no reason/emotion mind/body split. As the great Buddhist philosopher Nāgārjuna discovered two thousand years ago, nirvana (the other world) and samsara (the world of here and now) are one and the same. This is not to say that the neocortex is incapable of exerting control over the older parts of the brain—it is. Being a method of control is, essentially, what the many spiritual traditions were developed for. Keeping desire in check is one of the primary goals of meditation and prayer. But in Buddhism, the young monk is trained not to block out passions and desires, just to let them dissipate. To try and block them out only will ensure they will arise (echoing Jung's Shadow idea).

Like the Monkey King, Dionysus represents the wild and untamed that is a necessary source for creativity and freedom. Like most tricksters, he is a wanderer and shape-shifter, who indulges in the arts as well as the pleasures of living, though like all wild men he flirts with the underside, the Shadow, climbing into the valley of death. He is similar to the Egyptian Osiris, who was able to return from death to become the god of the dead, which in Trickster fashion is the story of survival, of life itself, able to resurrect from the ashes. In the Jesus Trickster stories (of course Jesus being another figure who conquers death), we see the Christ child as a trickster character in tales that go back as early as the second century. Jesus is portrayed as powerful and wise in some of the stories, while in others he is malevolent, in which case we see the reemergence of the dual nature of god—trickster—good and evil— found in most religious traditions around the world (ancient Christians would have recognized the naughty Jesus child in contemporary pagan stories of other deities whose early years were troublesome). The Jesus-child-as-Trickster tradition still continues in Latin America, where contemporary stories of the Christ child are still invented and told. While Trickster is usually a god, he still has limitations within his pantheon and cosmos, which are causes for frustration, and Trickster is also afflicted with the same cravings and desires as mortal men.

In some of these stories we also see Trickster as the rebel against power and authority. The Jesus child rebuffs his parents and the community, turning everything upside down. The Monkey King takes on the hosts of Heaven, and Prometheus battles with Zeus, stealing fire for the benefit of men. Pandora, like Eve, also resists the commands of the dominant god, because of her curiosity, a trickster trait, which implies a mind at work—not the automaton the gods often desire their creations to be. And of course it is Jesus in the Christian tradition who rebels against the Old Testament god by reinventing the ancient laws, even as he wanders into the desert to confront his demons.

It is this fierce wanting to know that drives tricksters from every culture to wander the earth, go into the desert, pry into things, and not be willing to accept the official party line. But the trickster's intelligence is usually not Intellectual; rather Trickster's smarts are emotive and intuitive. We see Isis as the trickster who dares go against Seth to put back her brother/husband from the fourteen pieces he has been cut into and scattered throughout Egypt; it's because of her emotional connection that she defies logic. Her incredible desire moves her to act. We see in We-gyet, an American Indian Trickster from the Northwest Coast acting emotionally.

In the Tar Baby, the most famous trickster story in North America, of African origins, we see how Bre'r Rabbit outsmarts Bre'r Fox, and in this he stands for the ways in which black people have been forced to outsmart white people. We see the same thing in the John stories (John being a reoccurring trickster character in African American folklore), with not only a satirical view of the white master, but of John as well, whose situation is one of privilege as a servant of the big house. Nevertheless, he is still a slave, and he uses all of his cunning to outwit the master, who would end John's life at the snap of a finger. Coyote represents the same force of survival for most Native Americans. Through slyness, cunning, and persistence, something of the traditional culture and of ethnic dignity survives. But in Japan, Tanuki, another animal trickster, is a little devil of a character, funny, but essentially mischievous without any good qualities—much as Coyote is for the Hopi in Arizona, while for the neighboring Navajo Coyote is an important god of their pantheon, central to the Coyote Way Healing Ceremonies. In Fox and Snake, we see the entire question of altruism being addressed, with the verdict being that if it does exist, it is not seen in these parts, which echoes a central problem in biology that Richard Dawkins mentioned in *The Selfish Genes*: How can an organism that wants to spread its own genes ever put itself at risk to be altruistic to another within its species? Overall, questions of ethics, justice, morality, fairness, and the nature of our species are addressed in these stories with a variety of responses relfecting the entire range of human morality: cruelty to love.

The Wonderful Tar Baby Story (African American)

"Didn't the fox never catch the rabbit, Uncle Remus?" asked the little boy the next evening.

"He come mighty nigh it, honey, sho's you born—Brer Fox did. One day atter Brer Rabbit fool 'im wid dat calamus root, Brer Fox went ter wuk en got 'im some tar, en mix it wid some turkentime, en fix up a contrapshun w'at he call a Tar-Baby, en he tuck dish yer Tar-Baby en he sot 'er in de big road, en den he lay off in de bushes fer to see what de news wuz gwine ter be. En he didn't hatter wait long, nudder, kaze bimeby here come Brer Rabbit pacin' down de road—lippity-clippity, clippity-lippity—dez ez sassy ez a jay-bird. Brer Fox, he lay low. Brer Rabbit come prancin' 'long twel he spy de Tar-Baby, en den he fotch up on his behime legs like he wuz 'stonished.

De Tar Baby, she sot dar, she did, en Brer Fox, he lay low.

"'Mawnin'!' sez Brer Rabbit, sezee—'nice wedder dis mawnin'" sezee.

"Tar-Baby ain't sayin' nuthin'," en Brer Fox he lay low.

"'How duz yo' sym'tums seem ter segashuate?' sez Brer Rabbit, sezee. "Brer Fox, he wink his eye slow, en lay low, en de Tar-Baby, she ain't sayin' nuthin'.

"'How you come on, den? Is you deaf?' sez Brer Rabbit, sezee. 'Kaze if you is, I kin holler louder,' sezee.

"Tar-Baby stay still, en Brer Fox, he lay low.

"'You er stuck up, dat's w'at you is,' says Brer Rabbit, sezee, 'en I;m gwine ter kyore you, dat's w'at I'm a gwine ter do,' sezee.

"Brer Fox, he sorter chuckle in his stummick, he did, but Tar-Baby ain't sayin' nothin'.

"'I'm gwine ter larn you how ter talk ter 'spectubble folks ef hit's de las' ack,' sez Brer Rabbit, sezee. 'Ef you don't take off dat hat en tell me howdy, I'm gwine ter bus' you wide open,' sezee.

"Tar-Baby stay still, en Brer Fox, he lay low.

"Brer Rabbit keep on axin' 'im, en de Tar-Baby, she keep on sayin' nothin', twel present'y Brer Rabbit draw back wid his fis', he did, en blip he tuck 'er side er de head. Right dar's whar he broke his merlasses jug.

His fis' stuck, en he can't pull loose. De tar hilt 'im. But Tar-Baby, she stay still, en Brer Fox, he lay low.

"'Ef you don't lemme loose, I'll knock you agin,' sez Brer Rabbit, sezee, en wid dat he fotch 'er a wipe wid de udder han', en dat stuck. Tar-Baby, she ain'y sayin' nuthin', en Brer Fox, he lay low.

"'Tu'n me loose, fo' I kick de natal stuffin' outen you,' sez Brer Rabbit, sezee, but de Tar-Baby, she ain't sayin' nuthin'. She des hilt on, en de Brer Rabbit lose de use er his feet in de same way. Brer Fox, he lay low.

Den Brer Rabbit squall out dat ef de Tar-Baby don't tu'n 'im loose he butt 'er cranksided. En den he butted, en his head got stuck. Den Brer Fox, he sa'ntered fort', lookin' dez ez innercent ez wunner yo' mammy's mockin'-birds.

"'Howdy, Brer Rabbit,' sez Brer Fox, sezee. 'You look sorter stuck up dis mawnin',' sezee, en den he rolled on de groun', en laft en laft twel he couldn't laff no mo'. 'I speck you'll take dinner wid me dis time, Brer Rabbit. I done laid in some calamus root, en I ain't gwineter take no skuse,' sez Brer Fox, sezee."

Here Uncle Remus paused, and drew a two-pound yam out of the ashes. "Did the fox eat the rabbit?" asked the little boy to whom the story had been told.

"Dat's all de fur de tale goes," replied the old man. "He mout, an den agin he moutent. Some say Judge B'ar come 'long en loosed 'im—some say he didn't. I hear Miss Sally callin'. You better run 'long."

How Mr. Rabbit Was Too Sharp for Mr. Fox

"Uncle Remus," said the little boy one evening, when he had found the old man with little or nothing to do, "did the fox kill and eat the rabbit when he caught him with the Tar-Baby?"

"Law, honey, ain't I tell you 'bout dat?" replied the old darkey, chuckling slyly. "I 'clar ter grashus I ought er tole you dat, but ole man Nod wuz ridin' on my eyelids twel a leetle mo'n I'd a dis'member'd my own name, en den on to dat here come yo' mammy hollerin' atter you.

"W'at I tell you w'en I fus' begin? I tole you Brer Rabbit wuz a monstus soon beas'; leas'ways dat's w'at I laid out fer ter tell you. Well, den, honey, don't you go en make no udder kalkalashuns, kaze in dem days Brer Rabbit en his fambly wuz at de head er de gang w'en enny racket *wuz en han', en dar dey stayed. 'Fo' you begins fer ter wipe yo' eyes 'bout Brer Rabbit, you wait en see wha'bouts Brer Rabbit gwineter fetch up at. But dat's needer yer ner dar.*

"*W'en Brer Fox fine Brer Rabbit mixt up wid de Tar-baby, he feel mighty good, en he roll on de groun' en laff. Bimeby he up'n say, sezee:*

"*'Well, I speck I got you dis time, Brer Rabbit,' sezee; 'maybe I ain't but I speck I is. You been runnin' 'roun' here sassin' atter me a mighty long time, but I speck you done come ter de een' er de row. You bin cur-rin' up yo' capers en bouncin' 'roun' in dis naberhood ontwel you come ter b'leeve yo'se'f de boss er de whole gang. En der youer allers some'rs whar you got no bixness,' ses Brer Fox, sezee. 'Who ax you fer ter come en strike up a 'quaintence wid dish yer Tar-Baby? En who stuck you up dar whar you iz?*

Nobody in de 'roun' worril. You des tuck en jam yo'se'f on dat Tar-Baby widout waitin' fer enny invite,' sez Brer Fox, sezee, 'en dar you is, en dar you'll stay twel I fixes up a bresh-pile and fires her up, kaze I'm gwinter bobbycue you dis day, sho,' sez Brer Fox, sezee.

"*Den Brer Rabbit talk mighty 'umble, "'I don't keer w'at you do wid me, Brer Fox,' sezee, 'so you don't fling me in dat brier-patch. Roas' me, Brer Fox,' sezee, 'but don't fling me in dat brier-patch,' sezee.*

"*'I ain't got no string,' sez Brer Fox, sezee, 'en now I speck I'll hatter drwon you,' sezee.*

"*'Drown me des ez deep es you please, Brer Fox," sez Brer Rabbit, sezee, 'but do don't fling me in dat brier-patch, 'sezee.*

"*'Dey ain't no water nigh,' sez Brer Fox, sezee, 'en now I speck I'll hatter skin you,' sezee.*

"*'Skin me, Brer Fox,' sez Brer Rabbit, sezee, 'snatch out my eyeballs, t'ar out my yeras by de roots, en cut off my legs,' sezee, 'but do please, Brer Fox, don't fling me in dat brier-patch,' sezee.*

"*Co'se Brer Fox wnater hurt Brer Rabbit bad ez he kin, so he cotch 'im by de behime legs en slung 'im right in de middle er de brierpatch. dar wuz a considerbul flutter whar Brer Rabbit struck de bushes, en Brer Fox sorter hang 'roun' fer ter see w'at wuz gwinter happen. Bimeby he hear somebody call im, en way up de hill he see Brer Rab-bit settin' crosslegged on a chinkapin log koamin' de pitch outen his har wid a chip. Den Brer Fox know dat he bin swop off mighty bad. Brer Rabbit wuz bleedzed fer ter fling back some er his sass, en he holler out: "'Bred en bawn in a brier-patch, Brer Fox--bred en bawn in a brier-patch!' en wid dat he skip out des ez lively as a cricket in de embers."[1]*

How the Wicked Tanuki Was Punished (Japan)

The tanuki is a raccoon-like mammal who is known as a Trickster in Japan, capable of shape-shifting and all kinds of mischief, ranging from comic to cruel.

All the animals in the forest had been hunted to extinction except for three: the tanuki, his fox spouse and their son. Tanuki and Fox were very smart and have avoided hunters, but eventually they had to come out of hiding and eat. Tanuki's plan was to pretend to be dead, have his wife, Fox, shape-shift into a human man, go to the village market and sell his "skin" and then escape (for tanukis were rare in Japan and their hides valuable). Fox did this, and the tanuki husband was sold for an excellent price. He was taken to a man's home and thrown in the corner of the house, went through the open window and ran back home. Tanuki and his family ate well for three days, but then they needed more money again.

"Now, it's my turn to play this trick," Fox said to her husband.

But the tanuki was evil, told the buyer that Fox, the tanuki's wife, was not really dead, and the man killed Fox the wife. Tanuki had done this, thinking now there would be more food for him and his son.

But the tanuki would not feed his son after all, and the son had to scrounge for food outside in the woods. Eventually, the son figured out that the evil tanuki had killed his mother one way or the other. The son also had magical powers, and he set a wager for his father:

"I will shape-shift," said the son, "and you see if you are powerful enough to detect who I am."

"I will wait at the bridge and discover you," the father said.

The son went to the bridge but did not shape-shift. Instead he hid. The King and his court and soldiers came by and the old father tanuki, who was on the bridge waiting, thought this had to be his son, having changed himself into a king.

The old tanuki attacked, but the soldiers grabbed him and threw him in the river where he drowned.

The son rejoiced and went back to the forest to live.[2]

Fox and Snake—Good Is Repaid With Evil (Venezuela)

A son waking with his father saw a snake pinned to the desert floor by a piece of wood and tried to help the snake get free, but the father yelled at him. The boy let the snake free anyhow, but the snake was going to bite the boy.

"How can you do this?" the father asked.

"Good is repaid with evil," the snake said, while a burro walking past agreed, saying that his master had turned him out after a life of work and quit feeding him. A horse stepping down the road also agreed. Snake was still going to bite the boy, but then a Fox came along, and the father bribed Fox saying that if he agreed with him and saved the boy the father would sneak Fox two plump chickens.

Fox, because of his eloquence, was able to convince the snake not to bite. The man took Fox home with him and the boy, told the boy's mother what had happened, and that two fat chickens should be stuffed in a sack for Fox. But the old lady stuffed the meanest dog they had into the sack, which Fox ran away with, saying to herself, "Good is repaid with evil" as she watched Fox disappear.[3]

Sun Wu-k'ung, The Monkey King (China)

The Monkey King story stems from the Buddhist monk, Hsuan-tsang's (born in 596) travels to India to bring back original Buddhist texts that could then be translated into Chinese. People loved this story, and it was eventually recreated in a 100-chapter "novel," *The Journey to the West*, which most scholars attribute to Wu Cheng-en. Wu-k'ung, whose name means Awake-to-Vacuity, is the Monkey King, a trickster of many powers who also studied with a master Taoist. The Monkey King finds out how to shape-shift, becoming a tree as well as seventy-two other possible forms, and has an ability to "cloud-somersault" over immense time distances. He commands an army of 47,000 monkeys. He says, "I am familiar with the magic of body concealment and the magic of displacement. I can find my way to Heaven or I can enter the Earth. I can walk past stone and metal without hindrance. Water cannot drown me, nor fire burn me."[4] He has supreme self-confidence, delusion, is a major egotist, constantly challenging the gods in Heaven, including the Buddha

(Tripitaka), who puts The Mountain of Five Phases on top of the Monkey King to keep him under wraps. When Hsuan-tsang starts his impossible trip to India to procure the Buddhist texts, the Buddha picks the Monkey King to protect Hsuan-tsang, for which the Monkey King is eventually granted Buddhahood for his service, and in this sense does follow the pattern described by Radin in analyzing the Winnebago Trickster myth, of Trickster turning into Cultural Hero. (But it is important to note that this is a literary text, not just a composite of oral literature, so from the beginning the writer had a particular trajectory in mind over the long course of 100 chapters in ways that folk stories usually do not.

Some scholars believe that Hanuman could actually have served as the antecedent for the character of the Monkey King. It is also interesting to note that Gerald Vizenor, a contemporary American Indian writer, who often writes of the Anishinaabe Trickster, sees a fellow Trickster in Monkey King in his novel *Griever: An American Monkey King in China*.

Dionysus (Greek)

Dionysus was the god of fertility, and patron of the arts, who invented wine. And like many tricksters he had two sides to his personality: bringing ecstasy or animalistic rage.

The Wanderings of Dionysus

A ship lay in a harbour; on a headland that overlooked the harbour a youth appeared. He wore a purple cloak; his hair was rich, dark, and flowing; his face was beautiful. The sailors on the ship thought that he must be a king's son, or a young king's brother. They were Tyrrhenian sea-rovers, and they knew that they could never be called to account for anything that they did in that place. So they made a plan to seize the youth and hold him for ransom, or else sell him into slavery in some far land.

They seized him and they brought him on board the ship in bonds. He did not cry out; he sat upon the deck with a smile on his lips and a gleam in his dark eyes. And when the helmsman looked upon him he cried out to his companions, "Madmen, why have ye done this? I tell you that the one whom you have bound is one of the Olympians! Come! Let us set him free at once! Do not have him turn his rage against us, or the winds and the sea may be stirred up against our ship. I tell you that not even our well-built ship can carry such a one as he!"

But the master of the ship laughed at the words of the helmsman. "Madman yourself," he said, "with your talk of Olympians!" He gave command to have the ship taken out of that harbour. Then to the helmsman he said, "Leave the business of dealing with our prize to us. Mark the wind, you, and help to hoist the sail. As for the youth we have taken, I know what kind of a fellow he is. He will say nothing; he will keep smiling there. But soon he will talk, I warrant you! He will tell us where his friends and his brothers are, and how much we are likely to get by way of ransom for him. Or else he will stand in the market-place until we find out what price he will fetch."

So the master of the sea-rovers spoke, and the mast went up; the sail was hoisted; the wind filled it, and the ship went over the sparkling sea. The sea-rovers sang, well content with all they had accomplished. Then, as they went here and there, making taut the sheets, they saw things that made them marvel. What was this that poured upon the deck, giving such fragrance? Could it be wine? Wine it was, and of a marvelous taste! Could that be fresh ivy that was spreading around the mast—ivy with dark-green leaves and berries? Could that be a vine that was growing along the sail—a vine with bunches of grapes growing from it? And what was this greenery that was garlanding the hole-pins? The sea-rovers marveled. Then, suddenly, their marveling was turned to affright. There was a lion on the ship—it was filled with his roarings. The sailors fled to where the helmsman was and they crowded about him. "Turn back—turn back the ship!" they cried. And then the lion sprang upon the master of the ship and seized him; the lion shook him and then flung him into the sea. The sailors waited for no more; they sprang into the sea, every man of them. The helmsman was about to spring into the sea after them. He looked around him; there was no lion there. He saw the youth they had taken aboard; the bonds were no longer upon him; there was a smile on his lips and in his dark eyes, and on his brow was a wreath of ivy rich with berries. The helmsman threw himself on the deck before him. "Take courage, man," said the youth, now known, indeed, for one of the Olympians. "The others have been changed to dolphins in the sea. You have found favour with me. And I am Dionysos whom Semele bore to Zeus."

He was that God who was so marvelously born. Zeus, lord of the thunder, had loved Semele, the daughter of King Kadmos. She had begged her lover to show himself to her in all the splendour of his god-head. Zeus came to her in his radiance; then Semele was smitten and consumed and the life went from her.

Zeus took her unborn child; opening his thigh he laid the unborn thing within and had the flesh sewn over it. The child was born from the thigh of Zeus upon Mount Nysa, in a secret place, remote from the presence of Hera, the spouse of Zeus. The nymphs of the mountain received the child from Zeus; they took him to their bosoms and reared him in the dells of Nysa. He was fed on ambrosia and nectar, the food of the Immortals. He grew up in an ivy-covered cave that was filled with the scent of flowers and of grapes.

He grew into a stripling; then he wandered through the wooded valleys of Mount Nysa, a wreath of ivy always upon his brow. The nymphs followed him, and the woods and valleys were filled with their outcries. A king who heard these outcries, who saw the ivy-crowned stripling and the nymphs following him with wands in their hands, became enraged at the sight. Lykourgos was that king's name. He had his men chase them, striking at the nymphs and at Dionysos with their heavy ox-goads. The nymphs flung their wands upon the ground and flew to the mountain-top. Dionysos went down to the seashore. As for Lykourgos, he was smitten with blindness; he did not stay long amongst men afterwards, for he was hated by the immortal Gods.

Now the ship with the faithful helmsman in charge of it brought Dionysos to the island of Naxos. There the daughter of King Minos, Ariadne, became his bride. He went to Egypt and was received with honor by the King of Egypt; he went to India and had his dwelling-place by the River Ganges. And everywhere he went he showed men how to grow the vine and how to make wine that gladdens hearts and liberates minds from their close-pressing cares.

And everywhere he went women followed him; they had a frenzied joy from being near him; they danced; they clashed cymbals; they kept up revels that were hidden from men. With trains of women attending him Dionysos turned back to the land he was born in. He went riding in a car that was drawn by leopards that the King of India had given him, and on his brow was a wreath of ivies and of vine-leaves.[5]

Prometheus (Greek)

Prometheus, whose name means "forethought," was wise and able to foretell the future and was on the side of human mortals, giving them fire.

Pandora (Greek)

In Greek mythology, Pandora was the first woman on earth, and like Eve in Genesis, her curiosity unleashes unforeseen turmoil. But like Eve, she shows curiosity and intelligence, daring to challenge the rules of the gods:

Zeus was irate that Prometheus had given humans fire, and in punishment he had a mortal woman created of unbelievable beauty who would lie and deceive. Pandora.

She was given a container that she was not allowed to open. But curiosity got the best of her, and when she opened the box, evil, sorrows, plagues, and misfortunes escaped. The only good thing at the bottom that was unleashed was Hope.

Orpheus (Greek)

Many were the minstrels who, in the early days of the world, went amongst men, telling them stories of the Gods, of their wars and their births, and of the beginning of things. Of all these minstrels none was so famous as Orpheus; none could tell truer things about the Gods; he himself was half divine, and there were some who said that he was in truth Apollo's son.

But a great grief came to Orpheus, a grief that stopped his singing and his playing upon the lyre. His young wife, Eurydike, was taken from him. One day, walking in the garden, she was bitten on the heel by a serpent; straightway she went down to the World of the Dead.

Then everything in this world was dark and bitter for the minstrel of the Gods; sleep would not come to him, and for him food had no taste. Then Orpheus said, "I will do that which no mortal has ever done before; I will do that which even the Immortals might shrink from doing; I will go down into the World of the Dead, and I will bring back to the living and to the light my bride, Eurydike."

Then Orpheus went on his way to the cavern, which goes down, down to the World of the Dead—the Cavern Tainaron. The trees showed him the way. As he went on, Orpheus played upon his lyre and sang; the trees heard his song and were moved by his grief, and with their arms and their heads they showed him the way to the deep, deep cavern named Tainaron.

Down, down, down by a winding path Orpheus went. He came at last to the great gate that opens upon the World of the Dead. And the silent guards who keep watch there for the Rulers of the Dead were astonished when they saw a living being coming towards them, and they would not let Orpheus approach the gate.

The minstrel took the lyre in his hands and played upon it. As he played, the silent watchers gathered around him, leaving the gate unguarded. And as he played the Rulers of the Dead came forth, Hades and Persephone, and listened to the words of the living man.

"The cause of my coming through the dark and fearful ways," sang Orpheus, "is to strive to gain a fairer fate for Eurydike, my bride. All that is above must come down to you at last, O Rulers of the most lasting World. But before her time has Eurydike been brought here. I have desired strength to endure her loss, but I cannot endure it. And I have come before you, Hades and Persephone, brought here by love."

When Orpheus said the name of love, Persephone, the queen of the dead, bowed her young head, and bearded Hades, the king, bowed his head also. Persephone remembered how Demeter, her mother, had sought her all through the world, and she remembered the touch of her mother's tears upon her face. And Hades remembered how his love for Persephone had led him to carry her away from the valley where she had been gathering flowers. Then Persephone stood aside, and Orpheus went through the gate and came amongst the dead.

Still upon his lyre he played. Tantalos—who for his crime had been condemned to stand up to his neck in water and yet never be able to assuage his thirst—Tantalos heard, and for a while did not strive to put his lips towards the water that ever flowed away from him; Sisyphos—who had been condemned to roll up a hill a stone that ever rolled back—Sisyphos heard the music that Orpheus played, and for a while he sat still upon his stone. Ixion, bound to a wheel, stopped its turning for a while; the vultures abandoned their torment of Tityos; the daughters of Danaos *ceased to fill their jars; even those dread ones, the Erinyes, who bring to the dead the memories of all their crimes and all their faults, had their cheeks wet with tears.*

In the throng of the newly-come dead Orpheus saw Eurydike. She looked upon her husband, but she had not the power to come near him. But slowly she came when Hades, the king, called her. Then with joy Orpheus took her hands.

It would be granted them—no mortal ever gained such privilege before—to leave, both together, the World of the Dead, and to abide for another space in the World of the Living. One condition there would be that on their way up neither Orpheus nor Eurydike should look back.

They went through the gate and came out amongst the watchers that are around the portals. These showed them the path that went up to the World of the Living. That way they went, Orpheus and Eurydike, he going before her.

Up and through the darkened ways they went, Orpheus knowing that Eurydike was behind him, but never looking back upon her. As he went his heart was filled with things to tell her—how the trees were blossoming in the garden she had left; how the water was sparkling in the fountain; how the doors of the house stood open; how they, sitting together, would watch the sunlight on the laurel bushes. All these things were in his heart to tell her who came behind him, silent and unseen.

And now they were nearing the place where the cavern opened on the world of the living. Orpheus looked up towards the light from the sky. Out of the opening of the cavern he went; he saw a white-winged bird fly by. He turned around and cried, "O Eurydike, look upon the world I have won you back to!"

He turned to say this to her. He saw her with her long dark hair and pale face. He held out his arms to clasp her. But in that instant she slipped back into the gloom of the cavern. And all he heard spoken was a single word, "Farewell!" Long, long had it taken Eurydike to climb so far, but in the moment of his turning around she had fallen back to her place amongst the dead. For Orpheus had looked back.

Back through the cavern Orpheus went again. Again he came before the watchers of the gate. But now he was not looked at nor listened to; hopeless, he had to return to the World of the Living.

The birds were his friends now, and the trees and the stones. The birds flew around him and mourned with him; the trees and stones often followed him, moved by the music of his lyre. But a savage band slew Orpheus and threw his severed head and his lyre into the River Hebrus. It is said by the poets that while they floated in midstream the lyre gave out some mournful notes, and the head of Orpheus answered the notes with song.

And now that he was no longer to be counted with the living, Orpheus went down to the World of the Dead, going down straightway. The silent watchers let him pass; he went amongst the dead, and he saw his Eurydike in the throng. Again they were together, Orpheus and Eurydike, and then the Erinyes could not torment with memories of crimes and faults.[6]

The Infancy Gospel of Thomas
(Apocrophy Gospel, 2nd Century)

Thought to have been written in the mid-second century, this apocryphal gospel contains numerous stories of Jesus before age twelve, in which he displays both good and bad Trickster-like qualities (here translated by Tony Burke from the earliest and best Greek sources while taking into consideration the Syriac, Old Latin, Georgian, and Ethiopic manuscripts).

The Great Childhood Deeds of our Lord and Saviour Jesus Christ

1 When the boy Jesus was five years old, he was playing at the ford of a rushing stream. And he gathered the disturbed water into pools and made them pure and excellent, commanding them by the character of his word alone and not by means of a deed.

2 Then, taking soft clay from the mud, he formed twelve sparrows. It was the Sabbath when he did these things, and many children were with him.

3 And a certain Jew, seeing the boy Jesus with the other children doing these things, went to his father Joseph and falsely accused the boy Jesus, saying that, on the Sabbath he made clay, which is not lawful, and fashioned twelve sparrows.

4 And Joseph came and rebuked him, saying, "Why are you doing these things on the Sabbath?" But Jesus, clapping his hands, commanded

the birds with a shout in front of everyone and said, "Go, take flight, and
remember me, living ones." And the sparrows, taking flight, went away
squawking.

5 *When the Pharisee saw this he was amazed and reported it to all*
his friends.

2:1 *And the son of Annas the scribe had come with Joseph. And taking*
a willow twig, he destroyed the pools and drained out the water which
Jesus had gathered together. And he dried up their gatherings.

2 *And Jesus, seeing what had happened, said to him, "Your fruit (shall*
be) without root and your shoot shall be dried up like a branch scorched
by a strong wind."

3 *And instantly that child withered.*

3 *While he was going from there with his father Joseph, a child run-*
ning tore into his shoulder. And Jesus said to him, "You shall no longer
go our way." And instantly he died. At once the people, seeing that he
was dead, cried out and said, "Where was this boy born that his word
becomes a deed?"

2 *When they saw what had happened the parents of the dead boy*
blamed his father Joseph, saying, "Because you have this boy you can-
not live with us in this village. If you wish to be here, teach him to bless
and not to curse."

4:1 *And Joseph said to Jesus, "Why do you say such things? They suf-*
fer and hate us." And the boy said to Joseph, "If the words of my Father
were not wise, he would not know how to instruct children." And again
he said, "If these were children of the bridal chamber, they would not
receive curses. These people shall receive their punishment." Instantly,
the ones accusing him were blinded.

2 *But Joseph became angry and took hold of his ear and pulled hard.*

3 *And Jesus said to him, "It is enough for you to seek me and to find*
me. You have acted foolishly."

5:1 *A teacher named Zacchaeus was standing listening to Jesus saying*
these things to his father and he said, "Oh wicked boy!"

2 *He said to Joseph, "Come, bring him, brother, so that he may learn*
to love those his own age, honour old age and revere elders, so that he
may acquire a desire to be among children, also teaching them in return."

3 *But Joseph said to the teacher, "Who is able to restrain this child*
and teach him? Do not consider him to be a small cross brother."

4 And the boy Jesus answered and said to the teacher, "These words which you have spoken, I am strange to them. For I am from outside of you, but I am within you on account of existing in this material excellence. But you, a man of the Law, do not know the Law." And he said to Joseph, "When you were born, I existed and was standing beside you so that, Father, you may be taught a teaching by me which no other knows nor is able to teach. And as for the cross of which you have spoken, he shall bear it, whose it is. For when I am greatly exalted, I shall lay aside whatever mixture I have of your race. For you do not know where you are from; I alone know truly when you were born, and how much time you have to remain here."

5 And those standing there were astonished and cried out aloud and said to him, "Oh, what a new and incredible wonder! Such words we have never known, not from the priests, nor the scribes, nor the Pharisees. Where is this boy from, who is five years old and says such things? Never have we seen such a thing."

6 The boy answered them and said, "Why are you so amazed? Moreover, why do you not believe that the things that I said to you are true? When you were born and your fathers and your fathers' fathers, I, who was created before this world, know accurately."

7 And all the people listening were speechless, no longer able to speak to him. Approaching them, he skipped about and said, "I was playing with you because I know you are amazed by trifles and to the wise you are small."[7]

Cakchiquel Maya (Guatemala)/Matias Sicajan

Jesus was in jail, and the guards thought he was smoking, as they noticed the tip of a lit cigar. But it was only a firefly. Jesus Christ was gone.[8]

We-Gyet ('Ksan, Northwest Coast)

We-gyet's fortunes had changed. He had found a wife who supplied him with all the food he could eat! We-gyet gorged and gorged on salmon, yet for every salmon he ate his busy wife hung two new ones on the drying racks. They had houses full of dried salmon. Whenever his wife went fishing salmon miraculously appeared at her feet.

This wife was not only busy, she was beautiful. Her flame-colored hair sparkled like those chips off the sun, the stars. We-gyet greatly admired this hair and wished his could be the same.

We-gyet's wife knew, without being told, that We-gyet wanted hair like hers. So because she was nax nok [supernatural, or able to read the mind of another] and because she loved the Big Man she had married, she gave We-gyet hair that gleamed like her own.

We-gyet was so happy! A good wife, a full stomach and radiant hair! What more could a man ask? His journeying seemed at an end.

One day, as he walked through the smokehouse, a drying humpback salmon caught in his hair.

Quick-tempered We-gyet tore the humpback off the drying bar on which it hung and flung the fish to the floor where it landed among the ashes.

As We-gyet did this, he spoke roughly to the salmon. "You of the big, ugly hump, how dare you disturb the order of my fine red hair. The ashes are too good for you, clumsy, careless one!"

Without saying a word, We-gyet's wife put down her cutting tool and left the house. She walked to the water. There, making a sound that was half whistle and half the moaning of the surf, she disappeared into the water.

When she gave her whistling call, the fish in the houses came to life and one by one they followed the red-headed woman into the water. They never came back.

As the fish disappeared, We-gyet's hair began to fall out. "Don't, hair! Don't, oh don't!" begged We-gyet. But the hair continued to fall. It lay on the ground in a pile. We-gyet picked it up and tried to replace it on his head but his own black, coarse hair had grown back. His own hair seemed very ugly indeed.

Too late We-gyet realized he had committed an unpardonable crime, he had broken the law that decreed that no one must speak roughly or rudely to a creature of nature. As a punishment, his good fortune, like his wife and his hair, had vanished. Sadly he journeyed on alone.[9]

⑰

THE TRICKSTER PERSONIFIED

The genius of clowning is transforming the little, everyday annoy-
ances, not only overcoming, but actually transforming them into
something strange and terrific . . . it is the power to extract mirth out
of nothing and less than nothing.

—"Grock" Karl Adrien

No one can possibly know when the first Trickster became incarnate,
turning into a living, breathing human being who acted out some of the
characteristics of the trickster of myth. Or maybe it was the other way
around—some real clownish character in some long-lost tribal society
was made immortal in a tale. But whatever it was, laughter had to be
the desired effect. Interestingly enough, laughter is not only a human
characteristic; it probably occurs throughout the world of mammals, and
is an old trait. According to Jaak Panksepp, a neuroscientist and psy-
chologist at Washington State University, "Laughter is an honest social
signal because it's hard to fake. We're dealing with something powerful,
ancient and crude. It's a kind of behavioral fossil showing the roots that
all human beings, maybe all mammals, have in common."[1] According to
the *New York Times*,

The human ha-ha evolved from the rhythmic sound—pant-pant—made
by primates like chimpanzees when they tickle and chase one another

while playing. . . . Panksepp thinks the brain has ancient wiring to produce laughter so that young animals learn to play with one another. The laughter stimulates euphoria circuits in the brain and also reassures the other animals that they're playing, not fighting. "Primal laughter evolved as a signaling device to highlight readiness for friendly interaction," Panksepp says. "Sophisticated social animals such as mammals need an emotionally positive mechanism to help create social brains and to weave organisms effectively into the social fabric." The link is most likely through play, which is one of the hallmarks of mammals. In play we see the constant give and take of mock challenge, mock stalking, chasing, fighting, and the repetition of other behaviors that will eventually add to a young mammals' arsenal for survival. In play, we see evidence of teasing and testing, the repetition of actions that somehow seem to translate (into our human perceptions) as fun.[2]

The notion that animals may have "fun" goes against the long-held prohibition against anthropomorphism, reading "human" thoughts and emotions into animal behavior, but that old paradigm no longer holds as we see that the same chemicals are being released in the brains of other mammals as they are in humans when activities we perceive as "fun" occur. The age-old antecedents for trickster-like behavior may be in the playful episode of a young monkey pulling its mother's tail, or of a wolf pup taking a food scrap from its mother and scurrying off—while fully aware that there is no escaping her. Even at this ancient stage of interplay between mother and offspring, we can see how elements of trickster-like behavior might have emerged: the testing of the adult world and all of its behavioral codes; for every kind of social animal has boundaries, rules defining social structure. P. D. MacLean states in "Brain Evolution Relating to Family, Play, and the Separation Call" that play might have originated as a method of bonding:

> Mammals stem from the mammal-like reptiles (therapsids) that were widely prevalent in Pangaea 250 million years ago. In the evolutionary transition from reptiles to mammals, three key developments were (1) nursing, in conjunction with maternal care; (2) audiovocal communication for maintaining maternal-offspring contact; and (3) play. The separation call perhaps ranks as the earliest and most basic mammalian vocalization, while play may have functioned originally to promote harmony in the nest. How did such family-related behavior develop? In its evolution,

the forebrain of advanced mammals has expanded as a triune structure that anatomically and chemically reflects ancestral commonalities with reptiles, early mammals, and late mammals. Recent findings suggest that the development of the behavioral triad in question may have depended on the evolution of the thalamocingulate division of the limbic system, a derivative from early mammals. The thalamocingulate division (which has no distinctive counterpart in the reptilian brain) is, in turn, geared in with the prefrontal neocortex that, in human beings, may be inferred to play a key role in familial acculturation.[3]

At some point, our hominid ancestors began to perform in certain "unusual" and "funny" attention-getting ways, and we can see elements of humorous behavior in chimps. Eventually, as we emerged into Homo sapiens, full-blown comedic trickster traits—singing, chanting, clowning, gesturing, clapping hands, pounding on a drum, telling a story, slapping on body adornments such as red mud, drawing on rocks, and dancing emerged, most likely (as we have seen) as part of the courting arts. Until the development of state-level societies the individuals who led or excelled in these activities would not have been seen as, nor would they have seen themselves as, "artists." For these "artistic" activities would have been in addition to the other roles within society these individuals would have had to perform, such as hunter, gatherer, tool and clothing maker, mother, father, aunt, uncle, cousin, and so on. As mentioned, in most primal societies there is no word for art. But with the development of state-level societies, specialization of work and development of class structures, certain individuals would be able to focus on artistic endeavors, including clowning.

With the development of writing, the encoding of myth into permanent texts necessarily meant that the role of storyteller and his or her relation to myth would change in some ways. For in societies in which the written word exists, it dominates as a source of authority, and no longer is it as likely that multiple versions of the same myth can be told with equal power, the way they are still told and thought of by preliterate peoples today.

Since writing was only the realm of the elite in ancient times, it was the elite who controlled texts. The upper echelons of ancient society, whether they were Egyptian, Greek, Babylonian, or Hebrew, controlled, to some degree, the production and transmission of myth, often incorporating themselves into parts of the mythic cycle. Hence, we have royalty as being thought of as no longer merely human, but gods, equal to the mythic gods that made the sun rise or brought death into the world. The priesthood became a separate caste as well, whose duty it was to help shape and maintain the mythic system, though sometimes revolts between the priesthood and nobility did occur (as in the case of the Egyptian pharaoh Akhenaton). Likewise, musicians and other entertainers, as well as all trades-people (military personnel, farmers, and artisans, who had arisen out of the earlier primal folk culture) began to specialize, some of them becoming "classical" players who were paid by the state for their services, while other performers remaining in the folk culture continued their folk traditions, making whatever living they could as players while still having to work in occupations. But for those involved in money economies, more of their time could be devoted to the development of their musical crafts, which coincides with the develop of more sophisticated musical instruments and musical forms in state-level societies. So, historically, there has been a split between those who could afford to live off of their talent, or wits (always a tiny minority associated with High Culture—classical), and those who maintained their artistic work while not depending upon it completely for their sustenance (Low Culture—folk).

With the division of labor, and the incorporation of myth into the governmental apparatus, the situation developed in state-level societies in which the personification of Good and Evil were often divided between deities, as can be seen in Zoroasterism, which influenced the other Mid-East religions. The trickster figure or god sometimes split into various disparate dimensions in state-level societies, while in primal societies the trickster tended to be merged with the godhead. Possibly this was done for political reasons, consciously or unconsciously, the authority of the state being challenged by the mythic notion of the good (which state-level societies always have in their interest to project) being mixed up with the bad. When the state is a theocracy, the dual nature of the gods can become a dangerous idea, leading to possible doubt and revolt, as the state is now the actual physical surrogate for the mythic gods. In addition, Trickster's personality is usually rebellious, by his nature wanting to overthrow elements of status and prestige. But the shadow of Trickster still haunted even the most powerful gods, who often continued to display trickster traits. Zeus, for instance, in Greek mythology, certainly retains his many trickster qualities. Having the god Pan exist alongside Zeus to perform many of the typical trickster functions such as sexual rapacity and musical seduction, did not mean that Zeus would become a benevolent figure. Of course, we see the same thing with Jehovah, who, regardless of the development of Satan (a Christian invention) still maintains his vengeful nature (floods, pestilence, war, and many other atrocities), even though Christianity attempted a wholesale revision of God into a personally caring and loving being. As we have seen in the apocryphal stories of Jesus, the Trickster element keeps emerging through the invention of new trickster tales. In theatric ritual we also see an overt acting out of the mythic stories, incorporating a variety of performance arts: dance, music, pantomime, costume, narrative, and song. In the pre-state-level folk cultures around the world trickster-like clowns arose as an important part of the religious calendar and social entertainment, and Trickster did not disappear with the advent of civilization as real people continued to portray the trickster persona.

For the flesh and blood people who have taken on the role of Trickster, there are always numerous forces at play behind their fate—family, education, religious training, economic status, as well as physical disabilities and general talents. It is often (though not always) the case that those coming from the lower to middle rungs of society are the ones who became the Trickster musicians, jesters, bards, or comedians (poverty and disabilities, for example, was a huge factor in many blacks taking up blues music in the Southern US). The "calling" to work in the Trickster trade certainly owed a good deal of its lure to attention and "success." Sometimes societies *required* one to become a jester or clown. Sometimes it was a preference, a calling, or it may have resulted from some psychic experience, physical illness, or a vision.

The heyoka of the Sioux was a sacred clown that a man was obliged to become if the Thunderbirds appeared in his vision. Lame Deer, a medicine man of the Ogallala Sioux (who I met in the early 1970s) says of the heyoka that

these Thunderbirds are part of the Great Spirit. Theirs is about the greatest power in the whole universe. It is the power of the hot and the cold clashing above the clouds. It is blue lightning from the sun. It is like atomic power. The thunder power protects and destroys. It is good and bad, the great winged power. We draw the lightning as a forked zigzag, because lightning branches out into a good and bad part . . . In our Indian belief, the clown has a power which comes from the thunder beings, not from the animals or the Earth. He has more power than the atom bomb, he could blow off the dome of the Capitol. Being a clown gives you honor, but also shame. It brings you power, but you have to pay for it.[4]

Steve Mizrach, in "Thunderbird and Trickster" explains further the link between the Thunderbird and the Trickster in Sioux culture:

Part of the link between heyoka and Thunderbird comes from Iktomi, the Trickster figure. Iktomi is said to be heyoka because he has seen and talked with Thunderbird. Iktomi is the first-born son of Inyan (rock), and is said to speak with rocks and stones. Like Coyote and other Trickster figures, Iktomi likes to pull pranks on people, but is just as often the victim of tricks and misfortunes. This makes him at once a culture hero, and a figure to be feared and avoided. Iktomi was thought to be a hypersexual predator, one who frequently pursued winchinchalas (young virgins) who bathed in streams, through various methods of deceit. Yet his pursuits and antics often wound up with him inadvertently getting hurt or winding up in trouble.[5]

The sacred clown is a Pan-American phenomenon, found in most Native American societies where the figure of the clown is an integral part of community ritual, the clowns usually acting as dancers who take on many trickster attributes, such as phallic play, obsession with food, and fascination with scatological behavior. The Zia clown/Trickster, "Ko shairi was the first man created and served as companion, jester and musician to the sun, and as mediator between the sun and the people."[6] The Zuni clowns were created when

there were two men and one woman, who were old and alone. The two children of the sun told them to make rubbings of their skin and to sing to it under cover. The being so created came to life as a boy and was never still. He was the first Newekwe and was always chattering, said the opposite of what he meant and disregarded all rules.[7]

Mud clowns, common amongst the Pueblo (and Navajo as well) are men smeared in mud, who perform and dance, sometimes with white stripes or other regalia, and in some cultures their job is to get others in the audience to participate in the dancing as well. The Pima-Maricopa "have at their harvest or Corn Festival men painted in alternating black and white stripes, wearing and carrying phalluses. After phallic play, they throw mud upon one another."[8] In California, among the Northwest Maidu and Southern Wintu, a person who is a clown holds that office for life, and his job is to "parody the speaker and burlesque the dancers."[9] The Pomo-Yuki clown is called an "ash-ghost," or ghost-impersonator, and they are the principal performers of their culture. "Sometimes these clowns prop open their eyelids with pegs and distort their cheeks with grass."[10] Clowns of the Northwest Coast, many tribes of which consisted of chiefdomships (having a hierarchical structure just below that of state-level societies), had clowns known as Fool Clowns, made up of people from the highest level societies, and their performances had to do with "ceremonial madness."[11] In some chiefdomship Northwest cultures, such as the Tsimshian, the chief had his own personal jester, much like the kings of Europe. Many Plains Indians had clowns, whose role was to act contrary, doing everything backwards (such as the heyoka), wearing odd clothing, and sometimes using whistles and dew-claw rattles. The Iroquois clowns of the False Face society in the Eastern United States acted in much the same way as the Plains Indian clowns. As Julian Haynes Steward says in *The Clown in Native North America*,

> the clown is nowhere among the American Indians purely a comedian. It might seem that since merry-making is usually his chief function, he should be chosen primarily for his comic talents. This is not so. Buffoonery is assigned to various organizations; occasionally the right to clown is even hereditary. The organizations and societies devoted to delight-making are primarily for curing, rain-making, wart-removing, etc. and only secondarily have the function of amusing.[12]

Steward goes on to cite the following as being universal traits of North American Indian clowns: the mocking of important ceremonies and persons; the breaking of societal taboos; comedy based upon sex and other bodily functions: such as scatology and gluttony. In addition there is a type of humor based upon "sickness, sorrow, misfortune, and need."[13]

> Red Elk, a contemporary medicine man, states than in American Indian cultures, there are both humorous and serious clowns. Serious clowns of the medicine society maintain the continuity of fertility, rain, crops,

health, and the various orders of Creation. They are the guardians of the ritual, ready with yucca plant lashes to catch a child and throw him in the river.

Whenever the clowns enter the stage of drama in a ritual and wherever they are found in the oral histories, stories, or songs, the clowns have something in common. Sacred clowns from different tribes can recognize another scared clown without word passing between them, they would be able to know who the other one was; what he represented and what he was placed on earth to do.

Early histories of oral tradition introduce the concept and the techniques of clowning. When clowns appear in the creation stories they play important roles during the emergence of "The People" into the present. Sacred clowns have a special relationship to the sun, almost like sons. Particularly in the southwest there is often more than one clown society. Example: Pueblos divide clowns into summer and winter clowns.

Clowns have several different aspects. Clowns are sometimes guides to the individuals whose dreams and visions take them to the World of Souls or the Land of the Dead. Clowns have a widespread association to water places such as mist, drizzle, rain, clouds, storms, steams, thunder and lightening. Clowns are mediators for rain.

One of the unique features of Native American sacred ways is the important place of humor and laughter in this aspect of "The People's" lives. Sacred clowns portray and symbolize aspects of the sacred in a special way, a way in which their teachings get through to us without even "thinking about" them. Clowns in their actions don't seem to care about concepts. They are not concerned about definitions but at the same time they define the concepts at the root of tribal cosmologies, the guidelines for moral and ethical behaviors, and the theories of balance and imbalance.

Clowns are the only ones who can "ask why" of dangerous subjects or "ask why" of those people who are specialists in advanced sacred knowledge. They ask in their backwards language, through their satire, and their fooling around. They ask the questions others would like to say; they say the things others are afraid to speak. Jokes, puns, and satire are forms of humor that are important teaching tools. By reading between the lines the audience is able to think about things not usually thought about or cause them to look at some things in a different aspect.

Clowns have an important role in terms of portraying and symbolizing concepts. Clowns portray the boundaries and the limits of the world by going beyond them, acting in a non-ordinary way while doing so, and in this way contrast they own contrary behavior with the orderly ritual directions and scared worlds. Clowns dramatize the powerful relationships. They show the dark side, the light side, they show us life is hard, and that life can be made easier. Sacred clowns integrate modern-day elements into aboriginal rituals keeping their dramas effective from year to year. Most obvious characteristics of sacred clowns is that they are full of contradictions. They have a mixture of innocence and wisdom, and they speak like "wise-priests."[14]

In *Black Elk Speaks*, Black Elk, a holy man of the Sioux who lived through the mid-1800s, through both the Battle of Little Bighorn and Wounded Knee, relates the following about the Heyoka ceremony:

> The manner of performing this duty is what is called in the ethnological reports a fool's impersonation. The actors in this ceremony are what the Sioux call heyoka—that is to say sacred fool or rather sacred comedian. Only those who have had visions of the west, that is to say of the Thunder-beings, can act as heyokas. The heyoka presents the truth of his vision through comic actions, the idea being that the people should be put in a happy, jolly frame of mind before the great truth is presented. When the vision comes from the west it comes in great terror, like a thunderstorm, but when the storm of [the] vision has passed the whole world is green and happy as a result. In the ceremony of the heyoka this order is reversed, the creation of the happy frame of mind in the people preceding the presentation of the truth.[15]

BUDDHIST CLOWNS

As can be seen by the above examples, Native American clowns encompass all of the attributes associated with the trickster of mythology, and we see similar occurrences in other parts of the world. In Southeast Asian cultures, mythic stories of Drukpa Kunley and Akhu Tonpa arose in the Buddhist tradition and are played out at public festivals. Drukpa Kunley, a Buddhist saint, (we have seen one story of him previously as Uncle Tompa) was a singer who taught through his songs:

> Finally Choje Drukpa Kunley arrived at Topa Tsewong's house, where his arrow had fallen, and stopped to piss against the wall.
> "What an enormous cock and balls he's got!" shouted someone watching children.

The Lama sang them this song:
"In blue cuckoo summertime your cock is long and your balls hang low;
In the purple stag wintertime the head of your penis grows long.
Throughout the year it's a long hungry beast,
But that is the difference between summer and winter!"[16]

As Steven Goodman says in an interview on Buddhist Tricksters,

> Drukpa Kunley and Akhu Tonpa, or Uncle Tonpa . . . are archetypal
> Trickster figures . . . [who] . . . teach liberation, usually by challenging
> holiness as a form of spiritual pride. If people are holding on too tightly
> to chastity, then they need a little prodding, they need some tickling,
> some humor. Remember, if a teaching is not threatening to the ego, the
> armored archetype within us, then it's not doing its job. So if people are
> fixated on chastity, a display of licentiousness will be useful. If someone
> thinks licentiousness is the path, then emphasize chastity. Sobriety,
> drunkenness. Logical thought, crazy thought.[17]

When Drukpa Kunley came to a pious community of worshippers, he
sang this to them:

> I bow to fornicators, discontented with their wives;
> I bow to crooked speech and lying talk;
> I bow to ungrateful children;
> I bow to wearers of cloth who break their vows;
> I bow to professors attached to their words;
> I bow to tramps who reject a home;
> I bow to the bums of insatiate whores.[18]

Like Jesus, this Buddhist singer includes even the lowest members of society into the elite, turning things on their head. According to Goodman,

> The mixture of the sacred and profane is common in Himalayan Bud-
> dhism. At festival time in Bhutan, people perform these sacred dances of
> enlightenment, and shadowing these very wonderful dances are Trickster
> figures called atsaras. They're slightly dangerous, untrustworthy jokers,
> and their role is to ape and mock the sacred dances at the same time the
> dances are going on. Often they will go into the audience and do rude
> things, such as dance around with a wooden phallus with a ceremonial
> scarf draped over it. The lesson is that it's healthy to invite all of us into

the dance, and every part of us as well. And it's very healthy to laugh. The
holy comes with a sense of humor.[19]

When we look closer, we see how prevalent Trickster is in the wisdom
literature of all people around the world, for it is often the case that
religious insight stems from that moment in which subjective and objective perceptions are shattered, and we enter a moment of paradox that
is shocking enough to waken the practicioner. The wisdom of the Fool
cuts through pontification and dogma, hierarchy, and all the kow-towing
to religious authority. Many times, it is only the Fool who recognizes
that idolatry consists of worshipping the messiah rather than trying to
become one—a Buddha or a Christ. For those who partake of praising
the deity, this seems heresy, but it is an integral understanding in the
"knowing" sects, the gnostic sects of many religious traditions. Hence,
we get a poem such as Shozan's, a Buddhist monk in the 1200s from
China rejecting even the Buddha:

> "No mind, no Buddha,"
> Disciples prattle.
> "Got skin, got marrow,"
> Well, goodbye to that.
> Beyond, peak glows on peak![20]

Likewise, the Four Great Statements of Chan (Chinese) Zen (Japanese)
Buddhism are summed up in Bodidharma's famous poem, attesting to
the fact that enlightenment cannot come from any outside source:

> Transmission outside doctrine,
> No dependencies on words,
> Pointing directly at the mind,
> Thus seeing oneself truly,
> Attaining Buddhahood.[21]

The Wudeng Huiyan (Compendium of Five Lamps) is a written record of dialogues between Chinese Buddhist monks of the "Chan" or
"meditation" (Japanese "Zen") school, composed by the monk Dachuan
Lingyin Puji in the early part of the thirteenth century that also stresses
how knowing cannot be transferred from texts, religious icons, or idols:
it must be experienced.

At one time, Danxia Tianran (739–824 AD) stayed at Wisdom Woods Temple. During some extremely cold weather, he took a wooden statue of Buddha and burned it in the fire to get warm. The Temple Director got extremely upset with Tianran and yelled, "Why are you burning my wooden Buddha?" Tianran pulled some burning embers from the fire and said, "I'm burning the Buddha to get the sacred relics from it." The Temple Director said, "How can a wooden Buddha have sacred relics?" Tianran said, "Well, if it doesn't have sacred relics, let's burn a couple more of them." The Temple Director was so upset that his eyebrows, eyelashes, and beard all fell out.[22]

We see the same mindset in Taoism, with Chuang-Tzu's statement:

> Where can I find a man who has forgotten words?
> I would like to have a word with him.[23]

The great American poet, Walt Whitman, said virtually the same thing in this passage from "Song for Occupations":

> We consider bibles and religions divine—I do not say
> they are not divine,
> I say they have all grown out of you, and may grow out
> of you still,
> It is not they who give the life, it is you who give the life,
> Leaves are not more shed from the trees, or trees from
> the earth, than they are shed out of you.[24]

Not relying on past textual truth, but looking at "things," is reminiscent of the same problem that occurred in the West over two thousand years after the Buddha began to teach—that split between the humanities and science (dealt with earlier)—with the humanities enmeshed in the truths of the written past while science was trying to break free of texts to observe the world as it is. A Zen saying—"If you understand, things are just as they are. If you do not understand, things are just as they are"—goes to the heart of bias, relating how our minds shape what we see, which in this jesterish comment makes clear the absurdity of dogma that would teach us that truth is fixed in a written form. Indeed, one of the basic tenets of Buddhism is that everything is in flux, which is very much akin to the scientist's conception that we must always be open to altering our concepts when evidence demands it.

What is sometimes called "crazy wisdom," or the "wisdom of the fool," is creative, protean. When Einstein said, "Imagination is more important than knowledge," this was the meaning. The Trickster's ability to jump out of line is the spark needed for insight or invention—not that the rational is abandoned—but there can be no creativity without a leap of the imagination, which often comes when we are not consciously thinking of anything at all. In the Zen tradition, enlightenment cannot come through desire or effort—as a matter of fact it often comes when doing the most simple tasks, like sweeping the floor or washing a dish. You can't study the process of enlightenment and become enlightened. Yet, you do have to prepare yourself, you have to be ready for getting there. And this is why the trickster wanders from place to place. In the Zen tradition, wandering with a knapsack on one's back is iconic—as the great Buddhist poets Basho and Issa often did. It is why the Monkey King took off for the West. And it is why in the tarot the Fool is depicted with a knapsack wandering into the daylight with a little dog at his side. Nearly all the North American Tricksters wander as well, and indeed many Trickster stories begin with the very words "Trickster wandered."

The trickster-like blues musicians of the South also wandered from town to town with guitars on their backs. It is searching while not searching, being there on the journey, and being open to what might happen, where lightning strikes. It is the allowance for possibility that allows the Fool to see what others cannot. And it is that ability to perceive even *craziness* as worthy that the greatest religious teachings as well some of our scientific insights have come from, everything from relativity, to quantum physics, to string theory, to parallel universes, where our intuitive day-to-day knowledge of how things should be no longer holds and we have to think anew.

In Zen education, koans have been used for generations by masters to prod their students to satori. The most famous of these in the West is "What is the sound of one hand clapping?" What most who hear this puzzle don't realize is there is no correct answer. This problem is meant to confuse the mind in such a way that the synapses are rearranged and one is forced to live outside the box. The following koans to live shows this:

> If you grasp the first word,
> You will realize the last word.
> The last word and the first word,
> These are not one word.[25]

> Not falling, not ignoring—
> A pair of mandarin ducks
> Alighting, bobbing, anywhere.[26]

JEWISH AND CHRISTIAN CLOWNS

In the Orthodox Christian tradition, Jesus says, "Seek and you shall find," but in the Gnostic gospel of St. Thomas he says, "Seek not and you shall find." It is in the second that we see the true contrary nature of Christ and the possibility for *knowing*. It is in the Gnostic tradition of Christianity, in *The Gospel of Thomas* (from the Nag Hammadi library, a text from the earliest era of the Christian tradition) that we find Jesus sounding very much like a Buddhist:

(02) Jesus says:
  (1) "The one who seeks should not cease seeking until he finds.
  (2) And when he finds, he will be dismayed.
  (3) And when he is dismayed, he will be astonished.
  (4) And he will be king over the All."

(03) Jesus says:
  (1) "If those who lead you say to you: 'Look, the kingdom is in the sky!' then the birds of the sky will precede you.
  (2) If they say to you: 'It is in the sea,' then the fishes will precede you.
  (3) Rather, the kingdom is inside of you, and outside of you."
  (4) "When you come to know yourselves, then you will be known, and you will realize that you are the children of the living Father.
  (5) But if you do not come to know yourselves, then you exist in poverty, and you are poverty."[27]

Jesus performed many tricksterish acts such as turning water into wine, multiplying the loaves and fishes, walking on water, raising the dead, and healing the blind and sick (sometimes using mud), casting out demons into swine, and he also used paradoxical statements that on the surface could made no sense. As Elizabeth-Anne Stewart says in *Jesus the Holy Fool*, this form of wordplay and wit was long a part of Jewish religious teaching:

> The obligation to study Scripture ceaselessly led to "a razor-sharpening of wits, to a verbal ease of articulation and to an unusual preoccupation with abstract ideas and speculation": in later centuries, this study also included the Mishna, the Talmud and the Midrash. Many riddles and folktales were thus passed on from generation to generation; rich in wit and irony, they offered answers to existential questions and insights into the spiritual life. For roughly twenty-five-hundred years, rabbis and sages have employed such material for didactic ends, for "by juxtaposing good with evil, light with shadow, grief with laughter, and honesty with sham, it achieves the harmonious unity of opposites that resides in objective truth."[28]

With Jesus there are numerous examples of him using parables that are paradoxical: "It is easier for a camel to go through the eye of a needle, than for a rich man to enter into the kingdom of God" (Matthew 19:24). "So the last shall be first, and the first last" (Matthew 20:16). "No one can see the kingdom of God unless he is born again" (John 3:1). The Sermon on the Mount, from Matthew, is full of statements that defy common sense in context of the cultural norms of the time:

> Ye have heard that it hath been said, "Thou shalt love thy neighbor, and hate thine enemy." But I say unto you, "Love your enemies, bless them that curse you, do good to them that hate you, and them which despitefully use you, persecute you, that ye may be the children of your Father which is in heaven; for he maketh his sun to rise on the evil and on the good, and sendeth rain on the just and on the unjust." For if ye love them which love you, what reward have ye? Do not even the publicans do the same? And if ye salute your brethren only, what do ye more than others? Do not even the publicans so? Be ye therefore perfect, even as your Father which is in heaven is perfect.

> Ye have heard that it hath been said, "An eye for an eye, and a tooth for a tooth." But I say unto you that ye resist not evil; but whosoever shall smite thee on thy right cheek, turn to him the other also. And if any man will sue thee at the law, and take away thy coat, let him have thy cloak also.

And whosoever shall compel thee to go a mile, go with him twain. Give to him that asketh thee, and from him that would borrow of thee turn not thou away.

In religious traditions around the world, the trickster character has brought a kind of backwards wisdom, that comes in around the corner instead of going through the front door, where authority awaits, asking for papers or a passport to enter. Trickster shows that it is the spirit of the law that matters, not the letter, which is exactly what Jesus shows in Mark when the Pharisees attack him and his followers for picking grains on the Sabbath: "The Sabbath was made for man, not man for the Sabbath" (Mark 2:27).

This tradition throughout the world of non-linear, internal knowledge, not dependent upon a priesthood or written literature, going against the grain of the everyday world, is often brought forth by prophets, teachers, and sacred clowns who exist outside society. At the same time, their strange pronouncements and revolutionary thoughts have been embraced, sometimes after the prophet's demise. The wisdom such philosophy imparts would seem to stem, from a scientific perspective, from the clash of conflicts in the brain where one self must emerge out of many disparate brain modules. In the wisdom traditions, it is the letting go of a fixed idea of self that leads to freedom and one's "original nature."

OTHER CLOWNS

In the Bushman religion the "trance dance is the central ritual . . . and defining institution," with accounts of these dances going back to the early 1800s, and attested to by "centuries old rock paintings in various parts of southern Africa that are replete with the trance motif. The deep trance phase is preceded by clowning acts of the dancers and non-dancers."[29] In Java, the *panakawan* is a clown central to Javanese theater who plays the role of servant to kings, or authority powers. The clown, Semar, is described by Kats this way: "He gives wise advice, showing more knowledge of the affairs and plans of the Gods than does his master. He not only enters the abode of the gods but himself appears as a god. . . . He is called blood kin to Hijang Goeroe (the highest god) and equal to Kresna."[30]

James L. Peacock writes that the

poignancy of Semar's power is expressed in the story of his death. Semar's master, Prince Ardjuna, has been bewitched by Shiva into promising to murder Semar. Though grieving over his obligation, Ardjuna still feels compelled to proceed with the act. Semar suggests that he ease Ardjuna's dilemma by simply burning himself. Semar builds a bonfire and stands in it, but instead of dying he turns into his godly form and defeats Shiva.

God though he is, Semar is still a clown, fat and grotesque, with female breasts. He speaks a gutter language rather than the refined language spoken by his master, and he injects uncouth and contemporary jokes into classical legends.

ISLAMIC CLOWN

In the Islamic world Mulla Nasrudin also teaches the congregation in the fool's way:

He went up to the front [of the congregation at the mosque] and asked, "Oh, people, do you know what I have come to tell you?" The crowd answered, "No." Nasrudin then said, "If you don't know what I have come to tell you, then you are too ignorant to understand what I was going to say." And he left the mosque. But the people knew he had great wisdom, so they invited him back the next week. This time when Nasrudin asked the congregation whether they knew what he was going to tell them, the crowd answered, "Yes." "Fine," said Nasrudin, "then I don't need to waste your time." And once again he left the mosque. But once again the people invited him back, thinking the next time they could convince him to talk. When he arrived the following week, Nasrudin again asked the congregation if they knew what he was going to tell them. This time, half of the people answered back. "Yes," and half of them answered back "No." "Fine," said Nasrudin, "Then those who know should tell those who don't know, and I will be on my way."[31]

JESTERS

In the folk culture of Europe, clowning and carnival were essential components of common people's lives throughout the Middle Ages, which included the Feast of the Fools and the Feast of the Ass. Humor was the anecdote to feudalism, aristocratic rule, religious proscription, pomposity, and political corruption. Mikhail Bahktin speaks of the way in which art elevated life in these clowning reversals:

> Because of their obvious sensuous character and their strong element of play, carnival images closely resemble certain artistic forms, mainly the spectacle . . . [and the spectacle] belongs to the borderline between art and life. In reality, it is life itself, but shaped according to a certain pattern of play.[32]

The court jester, which evolved separately in state-level societies throughout Europe, Asia, Middle and South America, and Africa, was the professional removed from the realm of the part-time folk performer, even though it was from the folk culture that he came. Court fools were often recruited from the ranks of skilled court musicians (as they often were in China) or from the streets or villages (where they were throughout Europe), wherever their abilities might have surfaced and been seen by someone in position of power who could give them employment. Their jobs were to make merry and to comment with great liberty, saying whatever came into their head, without usually getting his or her head cut off (Shakespeare calls the Fool in *Lear*—an "all licensed" fool, for it is the Fool, (as he dances, puns, and sings) alone among the court who can tell the King that *He* is the real fool.

Interestingly, the Chinese words for jester, such as changyou, also mean musician. In her book *Fools Are Everywhere*, Beatrice K. Otto relates case after case of just how the court jester, or fool, was given such license of commentary throughout the royal courts of Europe, Africa, and Asia, while using his musical and entertaining gifts to delight:

> Music provided one of the pools jester talent could be drawn from in both Europe and China and elsewhere. A description of a Ugandan jester at the turn of this century emphasizes his singing role: the " tomfool"—for Uganda, like the old European monarchies, always kept a jester—was made to sing in the gruff, hoarse, unnatural voice which he ever affects to maintain his character.[33]

This gruff voice also calls to mind the African penchant for altered vocalizations behind masks, resurrected in American blues music, which Louis Armstrong made famous through his singing style.

Throughout Europe "many entertainers were poet-singers, such as bards, skalds, and troubadours."[34] In addition, many individuals who played fools had some kind of physical handicap, such as a humpback, or they were dwarfs (many early blues musicians in American music were also handicapped, blindness being the primary affliction). And though the medieval fool of Europe was often associated with the devil (which the German proverb reiterates: "Where there is dancing and capering, there is the devil,"[35]) in Renaissance Europe, the cult of the fool was embraced, as in Erasmus's *Praise of Folly*, in which "Folly herself . . . takes the floor and mocks an audience of supposedly wise and eminent men."[36] In general, it has always been the role of the human fool or jester to do more than entertain, to also (like the Trickster of myth) turn the world upside down, showing that for all our intellectual advantages and developed hierarchies, deep down we are very mortal creatures for whom all the rank or money in the world cannot stop Death from laughing in our faces at the end. Indeed the portrait of death was "often depicted wearing the cap and bells of the jester" in medieval times "perhaps [according to Otto] to remind people that death has the last laugh over everybody and is the great equalizer."[37]

Enid Welsford's seminal work, *The Fool*, chronicles the long and detailed history of the jestering profession, with numerous accounts of individual people who took on that role in various societies throughout England, Europe, and Asia—from the Indian Vita "who resembles, though distantly, the parasite of the Greek drama . . . a poet skilled in the arts, especially music"—to the *fili*, "the arch-poet of Ireland in his feather mantle . . . with their 'musical branches' of little tinkling bells."[38] Welsford, in relating the psychological makeup of the people who became fools, says that there

> have always existed men who have a peculiar faculty for taking life easily, for gliding out of awkward situations which would baffle more serious-minded and responsible human beings. Such characters are a source of entertainment to their fellows, their company is welcome, good stories about them accumulate, and if they have little conscience and no shame they often manage to make a handsome profit out of their supposed irresponsibility. In a favourable environment such characters blossom abundantly and their way of life may even develop into a half-recognized profession.[39]

In the Tanali Rama stories from India, the Quevedo stories from Spain, and the Tyll Ulenspiegel stories from Germany, we see jesterism at work and learn something about people of wit who lived lives as real live fools within royal courts. These individuals became legendary, as stories are still told of these famous clowns hundreds of years after their death. The stories represent the Trickster's ability to stand up to the powerful with nothing more than a razor wit.

KANNADA; TAMIL; TELUGU (INDIA)

Tenali Raman was an actual jester of king Vijayanagura in Southern India in the sixteenth century, of whom numerous apocryphal and legendary stories are told in a variety of languages.

How Tanali Rama Became a Jester

In a village a very smart Brahman boy named Rama lived. A traveling sannyasi was taken in by the boy's looks and intelligence and told the boy that if he visited the goddess Kali's temple and recited a formula of words three million times, Kali will make herself manifest with her thousand faces and grant any wish.

The boy went to the temple, said the chant three million times, and indeed, Kali appeared. But immediately, the boy began laughing. No one had ever laughed at Kali before, and she was furious. "Why are you laughing at me?" she said.

"Dear Mother, when we catch a cold we have enough trouble wiping our nose with our two hands. You've got a thousand faces and only two hands, so what do you do when your noses begin to run."

The goddess was very angry. She said, "Since you made fun of me you are doomed to make a living as a vikatakavi, a jester:

"Oh, a vi-ka-ta-ka-vi! Wow! It reads vi-ka-ta-ka-vi whether you read it from right to left or from left to right," replied Rama.

The goddess was taken by Rama's insight, and her heart softened to the boy. "Ok, you'll be a vikatakavi, but your audience will be a king," she said and she vanished.

Tenali Rama began to make a living as jester to the king of Vijay-anagara.[40]

Tyll Ulenspiegel's Merry Prank (Germany)

Tyll Ulenspiegel was actually a real person, a "popular peasant jester . . . who lived in the fourteenth century." After his death a wealth of stories were created around him.

King Casimir had two court jesters of his own, and when he heard that Tyll was in the land asked him to come to the castle as well. The King loved his jesters, and he also liked to show off a trick himself. If the King argued with Tyll, Tyll had a quick comeback. One day, the King wanted to see which of the three jesters was the smartest.

Many nobles came to court. The King offered twenty gold pieces and a new coat to the jester who could make the best wish.

The first jester said that he wished that the heavens above were paper and the sea ink so he could make all the money he wanted.

The second jester said he wanted as many castles as there were stars.

When Tyll's turn came he said, "I would want the other two jesters to make out their wills declaring that their money go to me, and that Your Majesty order them immediately to the gallows!

Tyll won![41]

Quevedo and the King (Mexico)

The Trickster Quevedo, most important Trickster of Mexico, is based on the real human being Don Francisco de Quevedo y Villegas, a Spanish poet and satirist from the seventeen hundreds.

While Quevedo was in France, people complained to the King that Quevedo was obscene. The King called Quevedo in and said he had to flee from the country right away or be hanged because of his lack of civility.

"I'll be good, Quevedo said. "Another chance please!"

The King said ok, that he would allow Quevedo to play any trick on the King he wanted, so long as he demonstrated something (like an apology). Quevedo had three days, so Quevedo said that was fine.

The first and second days passed, but Quevedo could think of nothing. He didn't want to leave France, and he didn't want to get hanged. So he hid behind some curtains when the King arrived to receive the aristocrats, hear complaints, and give advice.

As the King passed in front of him, Quevedo put out his hands and grabbed the King by his balls.

Then the king yelled, "Quevedo! What is going on here?"

Quevedo said, "My Pardon, your Majesty, I thought it was the queen."[42]

Regardless of their professional or amateur status, the attributes of mythic tricksters have been incorporated into the persona of real human beings who have taken on the role of clown/fool jester. Like the trickster figure of mythology, these jester/fool/clowns could be both comedic and tragic, singers of both jigs and dirges. It is no accident that the skull Hamlet holds up in the graveyard is of the old jester on whose back, as a boy, young Hamlet used to ride. Trickster shocks us into recognition of our own mortality, shattering every pretension, every claim to nobility, showing that all of us will one day be eaten by worms. As the clown Feste at the end of Shakespeare's *Twelfth Night* makes clear, the journey from childhood through adulthood is a play that is soon over. The jester holds up his staff and sings:

> When that I was and a little tiny boy,
> With hey, ho, the wind and the rain,
> A foolish thing was but a toy,
> For the rain it raineth every day.
>
> But when I came to man's estate,
> With hey, ho, &c.
> 'Gainst knaves and thieves men shut their gate,
> For the rain, &c.
>
> But when I came, alas! to wive,
> With hey, ho, &c.
> By swaggering could I never thrive,
> For the rain, &c.
>
> But when I came unto my beds,
> With hey, ho, &c.
> With toss-pots still had drunken heads,
> For the rain, &c.
>
> A great while ago the world begun,
> With hey, ho, &c.
> But that's all one, our play is done,
> And we'll strive to please you every day.

18

BLUES AND COURTING TRICKSTERS

I've cried and worried, all night I've laid and groaned.
I've cried and worried, all night I've laid and groaned.
I used to weigh two hundred, now I'm down to skin and bones.

—Bessie Smith

The fact that the entire panoply of trickster-like traits keeps emerging in both literature and in the clowning figures of living people points to the fact that the same forces are continually at work in the human brain. But because trickster qualities are so aligned with sex and courtship it has been more difficult for Trickster to overtly emerge in Puritanical states. The often "coarse" nature of Trickster has not made him popular within Christian society who are always ready to see him as just another incarnation of the devil. Yet, trickster characters have by no means disappeared: they just go underground. This has certainly been true historically in the white communities of the US, less so in the African-American communities, while American Indian trickster tales are still told (though often in secret and at certain prescribed times). One part of the black community where Trickster has thrived is in the African-American world of the blues. Overall, in the arena of musical entertainment sexual freedom is played out in a much more conspicuous manner than the everyday world, and nowhere more so than in the music of the blues. There is a long-acknowledged relationship of this music to the carnal, and a long-time association of the blues with Trickster. As Brian Robertson says bluntly in the *Little Blues Book*, "Blues Ain't Nothing But Sex Misspelled."[1]

The blues originated as an amalgamation of musical styles that coalesced in some unknown black musician in the Southern United States, somewhere in the late 1800s, when he or she put together the basic twelve-bar blues progression. In the blues you can hear the poly-rhythms of African music, the call and response structure from African village life, the strain of Negro spirituals (themselves a combination of African harmonies, rhythms, and European musical scales and hymns), the story-telling tradition of Scotch-Irish ballads, work songs, and something of the Trickster-inspired tales of Africa (of which Bre'r Rabbit and John are both legacies). Since many blacks existed in a world apart from the rest of Puritanical America in the late 1800s through much of the 1900s, there was a greater allowance of liberty out of which the blues Trickster could emerge whose music and lyricism dealt mostly with sexual love. Of course, the blues is also intricately tied to gospel music, as the basic musical form developed in the musical tradition of the black churches. But blues took the devil's route away from the sacred, splitting much of the African-American community into two camps—those who loved the blues and those who thought it was a sure-fire way to hell. Unlike the tepid and romanticized popular music of white America, the blues exposed the rough and tumble rawness of real relationships that took place in a less than ideal world. For, even though slavery was over, which allowed the blues to develop and spread, America was still for most black people a terrorist state, where Jim Crow ruled. In the south the KKK was often in control. Reconstruction was an absolute failure, due to the government turning its back on the newly freed slaves, so many blacks lived lives of fear and torment, with thousands of lynchings occurring throughout the South, the most brutal butcheries imaginable—far more gruesome than most people conceive. These atrocities were often condoned by local law enforcement agencies and the lynchings themselves often turned into a macabre circus. Yet, even in this horrific state of affairs, black women and men were free to travel—and travel they did, with their guitars, banjos, and fiddles, as the blues spread rapidly throughout the South. Piano players, on the other hand, hopped trains and hitchhiked from one barrelhouse barroom to the next, city to city. This freedom of movement meant sexual freedom as well, which for black Americans coming out of slavery was something new. As Angela Y. Davis writes,

> The blues did not entirely escape the influences that shaped the role of romantic love in the popular songs of the dominant culture. Nevertheless, the incorporation of personal relationships into the blues has its own historical meanings and social and political resonances. Love was not represented as an idealized realm to which unfulfilled dreams of happiness were relegated. The historical African-American vision of individual sexual love linked it inextricably with possibilities of social freedom in the economic and political realms. Unfreedom during slavery involved, among other things, a prohibition of freely chosen, enduring family relationships. Because slaves were legally defined as commodities, women of childbearing age were valued in accordance with their breeding potential and were often forced to copulate with men—viewed as "bucks"—chosen by their owners for the sole purpose of producing valuable progeny. Moreover, direct sexual exploitation of African women by their white masters was a constant feature of slavery. What tenuous permanence in familial relationships the slaves did manage to construct was always subject to the whim of their masters and the potential profits to be reaped from sale. The suffering caused by forced ruptures of slave families has been abundantly documented.
>
> Given this context, it is understandable that the personal and sexual dimensions of freedom acquired an expansive importance, especially since the economic and political components of freedom were largely denied to black people in the aftermath of slavery. The focus on sexual love in blues music was thus quite different in meaning from the prevailing idealization of romantic love in mainstream popular music.[2]

While the common image of the blues is of men roaming the South, like Robert Johnson, thumbing for rides or hopping trains, it was actually black women of the classic blues period who first established the blues as a popular form and took it on the road. A common universal of all trickster mythology is traveling, which can be found from the Greek Trickster Hermes, to most all of the American Indian trickster stories. As Franchot Ballinger says in "Living Sideways," regarding Amerindian Tricksters that "we cannot deny that their wandering from their homes and from the rules—like their behavior in general—often smacks of hostility to ordered society and to its controls."[3] For black musicians having recently come out of the hell of slavery, to be foot-loose and fancy-free was the ultimate dream and an open affront to a white society that had kept African-Americans enslaved for hundreds of years.

One of the primary aspects of the Trickster figure is his liminal ability to exist between the cracks, to move in that space that is neither hither nor yonder, which African-Americans had done in many ways since they were first brought to America. The term "crossing-over" was used for light-skinned blacks who moved into the white community and passed for whites (as did a number of the black children of Thomas Jefferson and his slave Sally Hemings). Music itself was also a tool for crossing cultures in another sense, as from the beginning white people were drawn to the rhythms of black music. A remarkable folk drawing of Catherine's Market in New York City in 1820 shows a black man dancing for eels (a common occurrence at the Market), while another black man claps his hands, as a kneeling black youth watches. In the background is a large crowd of mostly white faces enjoying this spectacle, while three white men, two of whom are dressed in suits and top hats, lean toward the dancers, almost as if they desperately want to join in the fun. Another white man holds eels in his hand as an offering. The amazing thing about this drawing is the interaction between whites and blacks, an obvious coming together over music, which even in this crude drawing portrays such vibrancy you can almost feel the beat. As Lhamon Jr. interprets the scene, "These two performances, dancing and drawing, occupy one plane, pressed between shingle and roof. An incorporation of the participants into a shared event is going on here."[4] The jester-style entertainment provided by the black performers was tricksterish in that it opened up that liminal space. Obviously, it took decades, but such moments paved the way for a discourse that would eventually champion the cause of abolition and lead to the Civil War.

Most whites learned of black music from minstrel tradition, which started in the U.S. before the Civil War, bringing the sounds of African music to white America, even if the performers who presented it were white men in black face (wearing burnt cork or greasepaint on their faces to make them appear to be African-American). Women were not part of minstrel shows during this period. Nowadays, of course, minstrel shows are usually looked upon as crude and racist productions in which blacks were demeaned and caricatured, and there is no denying that the shows did that (some more than others) and that they were highly racist: but there is more to the story. The clown-like presentations of blacks was at times a double-play, inadvertently satirizing white society. The cakewalk, for example, which was a stock dance of the minstrel shows, had actually been developed by plantation blacks as a way of mocking whites' pretentious aristocratic mannerisms and dances.

Three stock characters developed in the first minstrel shows: "'Jim Crow' was the stereotypical carefree slave, 'Mr. Tambo' a joyous musician, and 'Zip Coon' a free black attempting to 'put on airs,' or rising above his station." Oddly enough, there was often real affection for black culture on the part of the actors and musicians who played in the minstrel shows. The most famous minstrel performer of the pre–Civil War era, Dan Emmet, who wrote "Dixie," as well as many other songs that have become part of the American folk songbook ("Old Dan Tucker," "Polly Wolly Doodle," "Turkey in the Straw,"), loved and studied the banjo (an African instrument) and greatly admired African-American music. He was also adamantly against the South in the Civil War. He regretted having written the South's theme song, "Dixie," a song he never dreamed would become an anthem for a cause he despised.

As awful as many aspects of the minstrel shows seem to us today, they actually were one of the first bridges between black and white cultures, for a great many whites fell in love with black music, even as racism against blacks persisted. After the Civil War the minstrel shows continued, but now they were performed exclusively by blacks, and for the first time—women. African Americans formed their own traveling troops, which allowed them their first opportunities in America to make a living solely through the arts. Even though the shows still portrayed comedic negative stereotypes, perpetuating the older minstrel traditions, these new minstrel shows allowed black men and women to move about the country, and the shows were not only popular with whites, *but with black audiences as well.* It was actually the blues women stars of the later minstrel shows who pioneered the classical blues tradition around the turn of the century, as the shows transitioned to something new. The blues women brought down the house, and the development of the Edison recording machines helped to propel their fame, as the record companies in New York found an eager black audience through "race records," targeted to African American audiences.

Ma Rainey was the first black woman to record the blues, with "Crazy Blues" in 1920, when she was thirty-seven years old. Ma, in her outlandish attire, personified Trickster and broke all the rules. In the words of blues historian Giles Oakley, Ma was

> an extraordinarily looking woman, ugly-attractive with a short, stubby body, big-featured face and a vividly painted mouth full of gold teeth; she would be loaded down with diamonds—in her ears, round her neck, in a tiara on her head, on her hands, everywhere. Beads and bangles mingled jingling with the frills on her expensive stage gowns. For a time her trademark was a fabulous necklace of gold coins . . . sometimes she wore a glittering beaded headband, and regularly swished a great big ostrich feather fan.[5]

For blacks, not long out of slavery, Ma's wealth and ostentation both mocked the pretension of white high society and culture while also allowing them to glimpse the possibility of wealth, for now a person of color had achieved that milestone. Ma Rainey sang, in trickster fashion, songs full of double entendre, where sex was the name of the game, as in the song, "Don't Fish in My Sea," part of which follows:

> My daddy come home this mornin', drunk as he could be
> My daddy come home this mornin', drunk as he could be
> I know my daddy's done gone bad on me
>
> He used to stay out late, now he don't come home at all
> He used to stay out late, now he don't come home at all
> Won't kiss me either
> I know there's another mule been kickin' in my stall
>
> If you don't like my ocean, don't fish in my sea
> Don't like my ocean, don't fish in my sea
> Stay out of my valley and let my mountain be[6]

As Angela Davis states, women such as Ma Rainey and Bessie Smith (who came on Ma's heels) "preached about sexual love, and in so doing they articulated a collective experience of freedom, giving voice to the most powerful evidence there was for many black people that slavery no longer existed." But even so, what these women were doing was not embraced by the overall black community. As mentioned before, much of the musicality of the blues, and its spirit, derived directly from the spiritual tradition of the black church and gospel music, but whereas the church choir sang for eternal salvation, the blues musicians sang about everything from sex to booze, from jealousy to domestic abuse, to cheating, hustling, and rambling: therefore blues was the devil's music.

The National Association of Colored Women, founded in 1896, chose for its motto: Lifting as We Climb. The lifting they were doing was to the middle class, and toward a vision of white values. This split in the black community also echoed the division that had long existed in the US because of skin color. In the United States, it had long been customary for light-skinned blacks to have greater access to economic potential, which went all the way back to the plantation days in which many so called "yellow" blacks were descended from the union of white masters raping or having sexual relationships with their black women slaves. Light-skinned blacks tended to be house servants, while darker blacks worked in the fields. Multiple divisions within the black community existed that were complicated and historically induced. (It should be noted that from the position of white society it had been law in many of the Southern states, that any person with even a drop of black blood was considered to be legally black).

As a performer, Ma Rainey flaunted her free sexual ways, which included lesbian relationships (another Trickster trait as we have seen—being bi or transsexual) which the song "Prove It on My Blues" proclaims:

> Went out last night, had a great big fight
> Everything seemed to go wrong
> I looked up, to my surprise
> The gal I had was gone
>
> Where she went, I don't know
> I mean to follow everywhere she goes
> Folks say I'm crooked, I didn't know where she took it
> I want the whole world to know

They said I do it, ain't nobody caught me
Sure got to prove it to me
Went out last night with a crowd of my friends
They must've been women, 'cause I don't like men

It's true I wear a collar and a tie
Make the wind blow all the while
'Cause they say I do it, ain't nobody caught me
They sure got to prove it on me

Wear my clothes just like a fan
Talk to the gals just like any old man
'Cause they say I do it, ain't nobody caught me
Sure got to prove it on me.[7]

Bessie Smith was even more outrageous, and was truly one of the great characters of American musical history. She too was a large woman, but taller than Rainey, and with a physical beauty Rainey did not have. Known as the "Empress of the Blues," Smith, like Rainey, dressed in feathers and gorgeous gowns. As blues critic Francis Davis says, "her heft was seen as evidence of an appetite for life that was essentially carnal,"[8] and many of the musicians who backed her up were said to have been in love with her. Like Rainey, Bessie Smith also swung both ways, sexually, and there were even rumors that she and Ma had had an affair. Wild stories about Smith abound, from sexual excesses, to single-handedly chasing away the KKK when they tried to disturb one of her shows. Smith, who grew up in Chattanooga in poverty and sang on the streets, returned there one time only after she was famous to perform:

> After her performance at the Liberty Theatre, Smith attended a party given by a friend, where she knocked down a drunken admirer who was pestering her. The would-be admirer then stabbed Smith, who chased him for several blocks before collapsing. She was taken to the hospital but returned to the stage the next night.[9]

Bessie also wrote and sang sexually charged material that dealt with love in a way that was a far cry from pop. In "Preachin' the Blues" Smith tackles her religious critics head on by suggesting quite clearly that the sexuality she sang of was also full of spiritual verve:

Down in Atlanta GA under the viaduct every day
Drinkin' corn and hollerin' hooray, pianos playin' til the break of day
But as I turned my head I loudly said
Preach them Blues, holler them Blues, let me convert your soul
Cause just a little spirit of the Blues tonight
Let me tell you, girls, if your man ain't treatin' you right
Let me till you, I don't mean no wrong
I will learn you something if you listen to this song
I ain't here to try to save your soul
Just want to teach you how to save your good jelly roll
Goin' on down the line a little further now, there's a many poor woman down
Read on down to chapter nine, women must learn how to take their time
Read on down to chapter ten, takin' other women, men, you are doin' a sin
Sing 'em, sing 'em, sing them Blues, let me convert your soul
Lord, one old sister by the name of Sister Green
Jumped up and done a shimmy you ain't never seen
Sing'em, sing'em, sing them Blues, let me convert your soul.[10]

Songs such as these have traditionally been seen, from the viewpoint of feminist criticism as saturated with sexual exploitation, the female blues singers themselves both victims and perpetrators of negative images involving women. The sexually laced songs where "taking your time" and "jelly roll" referred to women's sexual pleasure (according to this critique), were seen as demeaning to women, only serving to titillate male audiences. In addition, as in the song above, jealousy and hatred between women over the love of men is being addressed—which some feminists saw as doing nothing to strengthen the solidarity of women. But the blues lyrics are saying what evolution theory predicts: because of the nature of human pair-bonding, *women as well as men* compete for mates (rare in the animal world). But what was most lost on traditional feminists was the fact that the song is also a revolt against religious fundamentalism that did not allow for the sexual gratification of women.

Angela Davis, more than any other critic, has turned these ideas around, revealing the important historical role of the classic blues women in establishing strong feminist ideals. She states that such songs actually relate the "common fears and common interest" of women, through the sharing of stories of abusive men while sexuality itself, in all of its forms, is celebrated as something to be enjoyed (which most contemporary third-wave feminists now fully embrace).

When it comes to the relationship between sexuality and the blues for the male musicians, there is no new feminist critique to absolve them of pure, unadulterated sexism. While the male musicians of the next blues phase also had to deal with the overall problems of racism, the lyrics to their songs almost exclusively deal with finding sexual satisfaction from "a good woman." The other prevalent themes are traveling, confronting violence, and bemoaning the fact that they have been mistreated by women. Blind Lemon Jefferson, one of the first men to record the blues, sang "The Black Snake Blues" and "The Black Snake Moan," in which the snake, like in the Winnebago Trickster story, is the mischievous penis with its own mind:

> Um-u, black snake crawling in my room,
> Un-um, black snake crawling in my room,
> Yes, some pretty mama better get this black snake soon.[11]

The male blues musicians, instead of playing in "shows," tended to play on street corners, in juke-joints, honky-tonks, and rough barrelhouse bars, where fights could erupt any minute, and where whiskey and jealousies flowed freely. Stories abound of endless sexual liaisons that traveling bluesmen undertook with women they met in such joints which led to someone shooting them, poisoning them, or running them out of town.

Charlie Patton, a true trickster, described by one of his contemporaries as a "clowning man with a guitar," (who would put his guitar between his legs, behind his head, on the floor, while continuing to pick) is one of the earliest and most influential of the bluesmen and one who had a lifetime of difficult relationships with numerous women. As Giles Oakley says in *The Devil's Music*,

> The principal theme of the country blues, and probably all blues, is the sexual relationship. Almost all other themes, leaving town, train rides, work trouble, general dissatisfaction sooner or later reverts to the central concern. Most frequently the core of the relationship is seen as inherently unstable, transient, but with infinite scope for pleasure and exultation in success, or pain, and torment in failure. This gives the blues its tension and ambiguity, dealing simultaneously with togetherness and loneliness, communion and isolation, physical joy and emotional anguish.[12]

The cartoonist R. Crumb's excellent illustrated biography of Patton chronicles not only his genius as a blues innovator and stylist, but also his drinking, domestic abuse, and the string of brokenhearted women he left behind. Tommy Johnson, another wanderer, with a "succession of 'wives," is famous for his song "Canned Heat," in which he sings of his love for drinking cooking fuel, though he also consumed hair tonic, shoe polish and rubbing alcohol for a high. He is also famous for his mythic pact with the devil. (The rampant drinking and drug use of blues musicians is also reminiscent of the shamanistic tradition of altered states, which allow one to cross over into the other world.) Legend goes that Johnson makes a Faustian bargain with the devil at a crossroads: "If you want to learn to play anything you want to play and learn how to make songs yourself, you take your guitar and you go to where a crossroads is." "A big black man will walk up there [at the stroke of midnight] and take your guitar, and he'll tune it."[13] According to Francis Davis, this

> "big black man" was one of the many shapes assumed by an African deity called Esu by the Yoruba and Legba by the Dahomey, guardian of the crossroads, "the mystical barrier," as Henry Gates Jr., explains it, "that separates the divine from the profane world." A cosmic prankster, Esu/Legba "interprets the will of the gods to man and carries the desires of man to the gods." Gates notes that Christian missionaries to Africa made the mistake of confusing this Trickster with their own Satan. They weren't the only ones: in black Delta folklore, the literal crossroads formed by two highways or railroad lines was one of the areas in which African and Christian beliefs converged. Did Johnson's peers believe that Satan indeed owned his soul? No doubt some of them did. Johnson was a chronic alcoholic, whose songs . . . suggest he would swallow anything in a pinch. That he lived to be almost sixty in spite of these habits may have been taken by some, possibly including Johnson himself, as evidence of diabolical intervention . . . If instrumental prowess was part of what Tommy Johnson was hoping for in striking his Faustian bargain, he was tricked but good: his guitar technique was no better than rudimentary. But that voice—changing contour as it rises in pitch, it's the voice of a mesmerist, a master of disguise, a man both possessed and self-possessed, himself a Trickster.[14]

The falsetto voice employed by many bluesmen (as well as the guttural hollers [close to the style of Armstrong] and hoots), have an African antecedent. As mentioned, wearing of masks in African religious rituals, it was common that the actor would become possessed by spirits and speak in different voices, like the falsetto, behind the false front. Interestingly enough, American Indian Trickster clowns also "talk in funny voices like a falsetto."

The most famous of the country blues guitarists (also widely known for his falsetto singing style) who recorded later than Tommy, was Robert Johnson (no relation), who wrote the song "Crossroads," made famous by the Rolling Stones. Johnson was another traveling sexual rounder who was poisoned to death at the age of twenty-three by the boyfriend of one of his lovers. Legend has it that he also had made the same deal with the devil for his musical prowess as Tommy, at the crossroads. But as Elijah Wald, in *Escaping the Delta*, makes clear, telling such stories certainly did not mean that they were taken as gospel, for there was always tongue in cheek involved. Johnson's friend from school days, Willie Coffee said, "I never did think he's [Johnson] serious, because he'd always . . . come in with a lot of jive, cracking jokes like that. I never did believe it."[15] In John Hammond's documentary, In *Search for Robert Johnson*, he interviews an old girlfriend of Johnson's who "is quite adamant that Johnson sold his soul to the devil, but to Hammond's amusement she insists that the same is true of all blues singers."[16]

Of course, the devil that both Johnsons sold their soul to was the "devil" of the brain itself, in which language, music, and sexuality are all rolled into a related stream of neuroconnections that are the result of millions of years of evolution that the Trickster persona gives life to. Going through the stories of dozens of blues singers, similar stories of sexual proclivity and promiscuity arise, from Muddy Waters (and the many women he had relationships with simultaneously, even while married, even into old age) to contemporary players of today. One of Muddy's lovers in his late period of life was only nineteen, which is well documented in the PBS documentary *I Can't Be Satisfied*.

> I'm gonna say somethin' to you
> I don't care how you feel
> You just don't realize
> You got yourself a good deal
> She's nineteen years old
> And got ways just like a baby child
> Nothin' I can do to please her
> To make this young woman feel satisfied

I'm gonna say this to you
I don't care if you get mad
You about the prettiest little girl
That I ever had
She's nineteen years old
And got ways just like a baby child
Nothin' I can do to please her
To make this young woman feel satisfied
(What kind of woman is that?)

Can't ask her where she's going
She tells me where she's been
She starts a conversation
That don't have no end
She's nineteen years old
And got ways just like a baby child
Nothin' I can do to please her
Whoah, yeah!
Whoah, yeah!
Whoah, yeah!
To make this young woman feel satisfied[17]

This song is an exclamation of Trickster sexual prowess. Even as an old man, Muddy had to sing that he could conquer young women of child-bearing age.

Blues culture graphically illustrates the relationship between sex and music, but trickster aspects in musicians appear throughout the musical spectrum. The sexual exploits of rock and roll musicians are infamous, as are those in the world of jazz; yet, you could find similar stories in the less roller-coaster world of American folk music, just as you would in the politically conservative worlds of bluegrass and country (the last two of which are highly associated with devout evangelical Christian hymns and traditional values). In an interview with John Hartford, Bill Monroe, the father of bluegrass, admits that if he hadn't been a musician he probably wouldn't have gone through ten different women in his life. Even the staid halls of classical music are rife with sexual promiscuity. The contemporary classical world, as described in Blair Tindall's *Mozart in the Jungle: Sex, Drugs, and Classical Music* is rife with sexuality, and often involves trading of sexual favors for gigs and drugs. As Tindall puts it, in the early eighties, "everyone in the profession was swinging."[18] A similar story was told to me by a good friend who ran a regional symphony associated with a major university. My friend played host to many famous string players, including one august cellist in his eighties who had come to the University of Colorado to do a series of master workshops and a public performance. After the concert the master had two separate sexual propositions from female cello players (in their thirties) who played in the regional symphony. My friend witnessed (from aside) the master cellist turning down both offers, telling each of the women (without being sarcastic) that they were "too old."

This may all seem insane, but from an evolutionary vantage point, none of this is an aberration. The link between the arts and sexuality is deeply embedded in our genes, and we owe much of who we are as a species to that ancient connection. While audiences for music react in a deeply sexual way to music (recall how the brain releases the same chemicals for both), the relationship to sexuality doesn't just have to do with music. The connection exists throughout all the courting arts. Visual artists (look at Picasso's or Gaugin's lives of sexual conquest), poets, writers, and all of the professions in which courtship displays are a primary component (from politicians to teachers to preachers), have a certain propensity toward sexual promiscuity and trickster-like behavior. For these individuals are constantly, whether they know it or not, acting out courtship—sending signals that they are worthy to be mated with. Though males are more inclined toward multiple sexual liaisons than women, women are not immune. For remember, in our species, women also fiercely compete for men. The brain is wired in ways that generate trickster traits again and again in culture after culture, as we honestly come by (through evolution) all the confusions that continue to turn our lives upside-down.

19

TRICKSTER IN
WRITTEN LITERATURE

All my best thoughts were stolen by the ancients.

—Ralph Waldo Emerson

It is not only stories from the oral tradition but stories from the written literary tradition as well that testify to trickster-like patterns continually surfacing in the brain. From the moment oral stories were etched into clay, or written onto papyrus, the trickster figure emerged in literature. The oldest known written story (2800–2300 BCE) in which the author is identified is "The Exaltation of Inanna," written by Enheduanna, daughter of King Sargon, and a priestess of the Sumer-Akadian goddess Inanna. Her story regards her father, King Sargon, who as an infant is saved in a tricksterish act of deception when he is placed in a reed basket as a baby and sent down the river in order that his life might be saved (the antecedent of the Moses story). In Gilgamesh (2200 BCE) (Gilgamesh is Inanna's brother and friend in the first stories, her enemy in later ones) we have the first great epic (that also contains a telling of the biblical flood story that is much older than the version in Genesis). Gilgamesh himself is a trickster, as is his male friend Enkidu. (This story is the first known of the male-bonding stories that we see reinvented in everything from David and Jonathon in the Bible, Huck and Jim, the

Lone Ranger and Tonto, Batman and Robin, or even the Ambiguously Gay Duo from Saturday Night Live, all of whom in trickster fashion covertly touch upon a hint of homosexuality, which the societies they live in condemn.) Gilgamesh goes on his mythic journey to try and find a way to bring his friend back from the dead, confronting the power of the gods (he is half-god himself, as are many mythic personages who were influenced by him in mythic cultures throughout the Middle East, while in the end failing to reverse death and returning home.

Since Gilgamesh, the written literature of every culture is full of tricksters who continually appear and reappear in different guises. We find them in the writings of Chaucer, Shakespeare, Rabelais, Dante, Cervantes, (just to name a few), all the way into the present. We even see Trickster in the writings of Jane Austen—who (according to Audrey Bliger) employed the most "satirical commentary—to the indirect but more subversive form enacted by the female trickster character" . . . giving "voice to more radical views about the overthrow of sexism through the mouths of comic characters."[1]

"Nietzsche's prophet of the overman [Zarathustra] . . . [is also] a Trickster, since Nietzsche openly affirms the Trickster when he affirms laughter and joy," . . . [and as] Nietzsche also announced the "necessitation of the 'Fool's Cap'—something inherently Trickster and quixotic."[2] In the "picaresque" novel we also see Trickster as anti-hero, mocking all the norms of society. The word "picaresque" stems from *picaro* (Spanish, 1525), which means "low, vicious, deceitful, dishonorable and shameless" and stood initially for an actual character before it became associated with a literary one. Barbara A. Babcock, in "Liberty's a Whore," states that the term "picaresque novel" refers "in its broadest sense . . . to describe any first-person, episodic, on-the-road novel, and at times it is erroneously used as a synonym for plotless, formless, or structureless."[3] Babcock argues that rather than being formless, the societal codes that are "being broken" [in picaresque novels] are always "implicitly" indicated in the text, and that "the very act of deconstructing reconstructs and reaffirms the structure of romance." In such novels, the picaresque hero leaves society and enters the world outside of the civilized realm, learning to live by his wits and deceive; in doing so, the picaresque hero often moves toward a greater truth than society offers. This movement toward a "superior" alternative truth we have seen throughout the entire trickster tradition of the Wise Fool.

Since religious orthodoxy with its severe structural codes of obedience are the opposite of liberty, satirizing religion is usually central to picaresque literature. This is in line with most tricksters, who spoof religious piety, whether through American Indian clown ceremonies that often take place alongside the serious ceremonial processions, or the European Feast of Fools tradition in which a jackass was yearly brought right into the pulpit. We can see religion constantly being lampooned through American Tricksters of literature, like Huck Finn. In nineteenth-century American literature, the conman trickster was a literary figure who represented the shifting frontier and the opportunism that such lawless areas represented. *Huckleberry Finn* strikes at nearly every aspect of American culture: slavery, democratic freedom, Christian virtues, the rightness of law, and the claim that human decency stems from religious piety. At the same time we are presented with con artists of every stripe whose motivations are greed and self-interest, with only the slave Jim displaying thorough goodness, a complete altruistic spirit, though he himself is also a conman. But Jim must be. He has no choice in such a society, and by playing Trickster, whether in acting out the role of slave or "nigger," or "the dupe" (as when he gives in to Tom Sawyer's romantic proscriptions), Jim is able to survive, one of Trickster's greatest strengths. In today's tricksters we see religion lambasted through Bart Simpson, whose fundamentalist neighbors (the Flanders) are used to satirize the religious right, as well as through comedians like Bill Maher.

Trickster is resurrected in some form in every element of media: fiction, poetry, film, TV, cartoon strips—from Coyote and Road Runner to all of our television clowns and stand-up comedians to the slapstick of the Three Stooges, and the wit of the Marx brothers; from the comics of Doonesbury to Zora Neale Hurston's celebration of African American folklore tricksterism in her novels to Gerald Vizenor's new versions of American Indian tricksterism in his works; from Walt Whitman in his cry for sexual liberation to Allen Ginsberg and Kerouac, Thoreau, Gary Snyder. We also see trickster qualities in Michael Moore, Woody Guthrie, Pete Seeger, Bob Dylan, Bessie Smith, Bruce Springsteen, Little Richard, Billie Holiday, and countless other artists, where individuals have dared to come forth to speak truth to power in one way or another, while many have crossed the boundaries of conventional sexual and political practices as well. Even if some of these people became famous, and some rich, for their efforts, they *still* put their necks on the line, and for every one of them that are known and admired there are thousands of other artists who have evoked the trickster mystique while receiving nothing for it but the power of their own voices going forth.

Trickster may no longer be overtly recognized as a god in modern civilizations, but the spirit of Trickster is always there in the midst of us, as he/she comes out of our continually disjointed selves. As social animals, we have the contradictory needs of societal structure and release from the constraints society imposes upon us. That freedom is often obtained through play and mockery. Imagination and humor are the way out from being stuck in our mortal flesh, from being stuck in a world where only a few humans at the top control most of the wealth; from being stuck in a world where men control women; from being constrained by the wiring, hormones, and chemicals that go on creating our minds.

In Chaucer's (1342–1400) "The Wife of Bath" from *The Canterbury Tales* we see one of the oldest examples in English written literature of the female trickster. The Wife condones sexuality for women, as well as multiple marriages (five husbands), many hundreds of years before Women's Liberation came onto the scene. Not only does she wear scarlet stockings, but she has a "space" between her teeth (an ancient symbol for sexual proclivity). In the prologue, she gives an "apology" for her lifestyle, through which, as we read between the lines, we understand she has no remorse, no shame over. She revels in flaunting conventions, as she celebrates sexuality and even castigates her culture's obsession with virginity:

1 "Experience, though noon auctoritee
"Experience, though no written authority
2 Were in this world, is right ynogh for me
Were in this world, is good enough for me
3 To speke of wo that is in mariage;
To speak of the woe that is in marriage;
4 For, lordynges, sith I twelve yeer was of age,
For, gentlemen, since I was twelve years of age,
5 Thonked be God that is eterne on lyve,
Thanked be God who is eternally alive,
6 Housbondes at chirche dore I have had fyve —
I have had five husbands at the church door —[4]

But when it comes to a body of literature written by one person, in which Trickster dominates, Shakespeare is foremost. His many fool characters are at the very heart of his plays—his clowns and jesters telling the truth when no other character will dare, all the while making a mockery of official conventions, whether those conventions be marriage, aristocratic structure, warfare, or the madness of love. The Fool in Lear speaks truth to power when he says to the King

> Yes indeed. Thou wouldst make a good fool.
> If thou wert my fool, nuncle,
> I'd have thee beaten for being old before thy time.
> Thou shouldst not have been old till thou hadst been wise.

And the Fool continues the Trickster's tradition of sexual puns when he speaks of the penis, penetration, and castration, evoking Lear's own metaphorical self-neutering:

> She that's a maid now, and laughs at my departure,
> Shall not be a maid long, unless things be cut shorter.

In truth, it's hard to find any piece of literature that doesn't exhibit *some* aspect of the trickster figure, for it is the nature of writing to confront the status quo. Mikhail Bakhtin sees the novel itself stemming from the "current of decentralizing, centrifugal forces"[5] found in the Trickster motif: jester, clown, fool. Desire motivates every trickster tale, and desire is the driving force of all fiction. In American literature this craving often leads to physical wandering. From Huck lighting out for the territory to Janie's hitting the road with Tea Cake in *Their Eyes Were Watching God*, to Tom Joad and the Oakies in *Grapes of Wrath* trekking to California, to Kerouac's ramblings around the country in *On the Road*, our literature is full of Trickster's yearning, traveling, and desiring of something more.

Many fiction writers have also resurrected traditional trickster figures from their varied cultures, placing them into their stories and novels,. Though traditional trickster tales may suffer from a dearth of women tricksters (Trickstars), the literature of contemporary ethnic writers has seen them prosper. Trickstar has been embraced as a central figure in both fiction and poetry by American Indian women writers such Joy Harjo, Leslie Marmon Silko, Louise Erdrich; African American writers, such as Toni Morrison; and Chinese writers, such as Maxine Hong Kingston. Each of these women writers works with trickster mythology, reinterpreting ancient forms while developing new literary Tricksters. Then again, it is not only contemporary ethnic women writers who have embraced Trickster. Trickster has emerged as a dominant motif, symbolizing cunning and survival in a world surrounded by European values for male ethnic writers as well, from African American writers such as Ralph Ellison to American Indian writers such as Gerald Vizenor, Simon Ortiz, Ray Young Bear, James Welch, D'Arcy McNickle, N. Scott Momaday, Sherman Alexie, and others who have used Trickster as a way to spring out of the racial traps and reshape the boundaries of American thought.

20

TRICKSTER WAS WANDERING

And precisely because we are at bottom grave and serious human beings and more weights than human beings, nothing does us as much good as the fool's cap: we need it against ourselves—we need all exuberant, floating, dancing, mocking, childish and blissful art lest we lose that freedom over things that our ideal demands of us.

—Nietzsche

Looking at the few primal people left in the world, and looking at the records of those native peoples who have been studied by anthropologists and ethnographers over the last century, it's clear that humans everywhere have recognized contradiction as an essential part of human life. While some cultural groups, like the Puritans, have tried to reimagine human behavior in black and white terms, eliminating shades of gray (the shade where most of us live), the trickster tradition is one of embracing all human experience, recognizing that our conflicting desires (born from the klutzy construction of our physical brains) are also essential to making us who we are.

This philosophy of inclusion was put well by the Sioux/Lakota holy man Lame Deer, who I happened to meet at a Sundance in Green Grass, South Dakota in the early seventies, along with the equally fascinating medicine man, Pete Catches. At that time, a number of us white college-age students had been captivated by philosophies of American Indian cultures, and at NIU, where I was attending college, we had set up a drive to bring food and clothing to the Pine Ridge reservation during the onslaught at Wounded Knee (that second one where Nixon was in charge, right after the Vietnam War). One day, we were invited by Selo Black Crow, another Sioux holy man, to go up to Green Grass, where the original sacred pipe, brought from the White Buffalo Calf Maiden, was housed. Since the world seemed to be in a particular state of crisis, the sacred pipe was being brought out, for the first time in decades, as an act of healing. We young white kids were driving up to the sacred Sundance grounds, when someone in the car accidentally (in Trickster fashion) hit the horn, so we introduced ourselves in a less than sacred way; yet, we were given the honor of feeding the people by cutting up the cow and buffalo someone had brought in, and putting it into the individual pots of the women who came forward to receive the food. Shortly after, the camp was full of meat drying on tent-poles (to make pemmican) in the summer sun with flies buzzing ferociously all around.

Lame Deer's story had already been published by this time in his and Erdoes's book *Lame Deer, Seeker of Visions*, so to us he was quite a celebrity. On the grounds of the Sundance he certainly seemed one of the most important medicine men to the other Indian people gathered there. Speaking of being a medicine man, Lame Deer said:

> A medicine man shouldn't be a saint. He should experience and feel all the ups and downs, the despair and joy, the magic, and the reality, the courage and the fear, of his people. He should be able to sink as low as a bug, or soar as high as an eagle. Unless he can experience both, he is no good as a medicine man. . . . You can't get so stuck up, so inhuman that you want to be pure, your soul wrapped up in a plastic bag, all the time. You have to be God and the devil, both of them. Being a good medicine man means being right in the midst of turmoil, not shielding yourself from it. It means experiencing life in all its phases. It means not being afraid of cutting up and playing the fool now and then. That's sacred too. Nature, the Great Spirit—they are not perfect. The world couldn't stand that perfection. The spirit has a good side and a bad side. Sometimes the bad side gives me more knowledge than the good side.[1]

This is, in essence, the story of Trickster: the recognition and acceptance of our internal conflicts. Primal people often saw humor as the tool with which to address our disparate selves. Mark Twain said, "Everything human is pathetic. The secret source of humor itself is not joy but sorrow. There is no humor in heaven." What makes us pathetic, conflicted, contrary, depressed, and elated, are the very brains we carry, which came from the long process of evolution. Humor is one way the brain tricks itself into handling internal conflict and releasing tension. Humor, which probably started as another courtship art also became our way of handling the absurdities of life.

Like people today, our ancient ancestors must have seen life as both comic and tragic, for early humans with large brains had to have recognized that there *is* great wonderment in living: communing with family, having sexual relations, having children, experiencing love, experiencing consciousness, creating tools, music, art, ritual; enjoying the deep satisfaction that comes from maintaining one's existence through daily activity—the gathering of plants, hunting, and everything that goes along with successful survival; blossoming cultural development, and the beauty of the natural world. In other words—the joy of life. Likewise, they also must have recognized that as magnificent as life can be, our existence is, and always has been, precarious. For our world is perilous, and not just from the wild animals, parasites, and difficult environmental conditions our species has had to face. Rules, like avoidance procedures, were created long before written law because we humans can drive each other crazy. Religious traditions developed as well, in part, as another mechanism to keep things in check, while from the biological perspective the conscience evolved as part of the mind to regulate impulses that could lead to social disruption.

In a world where death can strike at any moment—where suffering can become one's lot in an instant, where infection can creep in through something as simple as a thorn piercing the foot, or a mangled code in the DNA, or a neighbor hitting you over the head because they think you're a witch—people have tried what they could to gain control. For eons, this meant trying to establish cause and effect explanations and pinning most of the blame on very human gods or on ourselves for not obeying them. Hence, we received such notions as Augustine's doctrine of original sin, which states that human beings, *and nature itself*, are corrupt because of Adam. Through such rationalizations humans have tried to explain the existence of evil. In *Adam, Eve, and the Serpent,* Elaine Pagels speaks of the cross-cultural ubiquity of attaching such blame:

> interpretations of suffering as the result of sin are by no means limited to Christianity. . . . Jewish tradition has interpreted personal tragedy similarly, attributing, for example, the sudden death of an infant to the demon Lilith, to whose malevolence the child's parents had made themselves susceptible either through the husband's infidelity or the wife's insubordination. Some rabbis of ancient times would explain, too, to a young widow that she herself caused her husband's sudden heart attack by neglecting ritual regulations concerning the timing of intercourse. . . . A Hopi child is bitten by a poisonous spider while playing near its hole. As the boy hovers between life and death, the medicine man learns that the boy's father has neglected to prepare ritual ornaments for Spider Woman, the tribe's protector, which, he proclaims, has brought on his son's illness.[2]

Everything from tsunamis to disease have been ascribed to human-like agency—such as witchcraft, or failure to follow societal precepts. Only science has allowed us to see past such ways of thinking.

Nature is not perfect and evolution never has a goal. The process is messy and often leaves us with unwanted vestiges, such as tailbones, wisdom teeth, appendixes, bad backs, fallen arches, the tendency to choke, and the propensity for female death resulting from impossibly small birth canals due to our walking upright. We have numerous mental vestiges as well. We come by our conflicted selves honestly. But whereas much religious orthodoxy would have us whipped and sent to the stocks for breaking codes of conduct—for even thinking of mischief—the trickster tradition, *which is also religious*, laughs at the realization that we are animals who live with animalistic desires. Regardless of our forks and spoons, we still must masticate our food, digest it, and expel waste in the end. Trickster doesn't let us hide from such facts. Trickster forces us to admit our "lower" origins, and thereby serves a central function: awakening us to our own pomposity by exposing us as sophisticated frauds. Trickster reveals our selfish genes, the most primitive parts of the brain; our contradictory brain modules, our obsession with hierarchy and status, our constant desire for food and sex. Yet, Trickster also allows us a way out by revealing the truth, bringing the totality of ourselves into the light of day. For we, like Trickster, also have protean abilities—we *can* do the unexpected. For even though we are biological creatures, we are not automatons. Trickster also shows that our sense of ethics is deep, and while we are capable of the most base behaviors we are also capable of intelligence, empathy, and love.

NOTES

CHAPTER 2: THE SILVER TONGUED DEVIL

1. E. F. Edinger, *The Creation of Consciousness: Jung's Myth for Modern Man* (Toronto, ON: Inner City Books, 1984).

2. G. Boeree, "Introduction to C. G. Jung," (UK: Archetypes, 1997).

3. Boeree, "Introduction."

4. F. C. Crews, *Follies of the Wise: Dissenting Essays* (Berkeley, CA: Shoemaker and Hoard, 2006), 247.

5. J. Campbell, *"Mythic Reflections: Thoughts on Myth, Spirit, and Our Times: An Interview with Joseph Campbell,"* edited by Tom Collins, *The New Story* 52, no. 12 (Winter 1985).

6. M. Groden, and M. Kreiswirth, *The Johns Hopkins Guide to Literary Theory and Criticism* (Baltimore: Johns Hopkins University Press, 1994), 403.

7. N. Frye, *The Stubborn Structure: Essays on Criticism and Society* (Ithaca: Cornell University Press, 1970),102.

8. E. O. Wilson, *Consilience* (New York: Knopf, 1998),167.

9. J. Gottschall, and D. S. Wilson, *The Literary Animal: Evolution and the Nature of Narrative* (Chicago: Northwestern University Press, 2005), 1.

10. E. O. Wilson, *Consilience* (New York: Knopf, 1998), 200.

11. W. J. Hynes, and W. G. Doty, *Mythical Trickster Figures: Contours, Contexts, and Criticisms* (Tuscaloosa: University of Alabama Press, 1993), 176.

12. P. C. Hogan, *The Mind and Its Stories: Narrative Universals and Human Emotion* (Cambridge: Cambridge University Press, 2003), 9.

13. E. O. Wilson, *Consilience* (New York: Knopf, 1998), 167.

14. S. Pinker, *The Blank Slate* (New York: Viking, 2002), 5.

15. A. Synnott, "Tomb, Temple, Machine and Self: The Social Construction of the Body." *The British Journal of Sociology* 43, no. 1 (1992): 79–110.

16. S. J. Gould, *The Hedgehog, the Fox, and the Magister's Pox: Mending the Gap between Science and the Humanities* (London: Jonathan Cape, 2003), 39.

17. P. G. Allen, *The Sacred Hoop: Recovering the Feminine in American Indian Traditions: With a New Preface* (Boston: Beacon Press, 1992), 214.

18. J. Gottschall, and D. S. Wilson, *The Literary Animal: Evolution and the Nature of Narrative* (Evanston: Northwestern University Press, 2005), xxx.

19. L. Osborne, "A Linguistic Big Bang," *New York Times* 24 (1999).

20. D. Evans, "From Lacan to Darwin" in Gottschall and Wilson's *The Literary Animal* (Evanston: Northwestern University Press, 2005), 50.

21. M. Turner, *The Literary Mind: The Origins of Thought and Language* (Oxford: Oxford University Press, 1998), 16.

22. L. Carroll, *Alice in Wonderland*.

23. V. S. Ramachandran, *The Tell-Tale Brain*. (New York: W.W. Norton, 2011), 43.

CHAPTER 3: THE TRICKSTERISH BRAIN

1. R. Kurzban, *Why Everyone Else Is a Hypocrite: Evolution and the Modular Mind*. (Princeton: Princeton University Press, 2010), 50.

2. D. J. Linden, *The Accidental Mind* (Cambridge: Belknap Press of Harvard University Press, 2007).

3. J. Ruddy. *The Neurobiology of Learning and Memory* (Sunderland, MA: Sinauer Inc., 2008), 9.

4. D. O. Hebb, *The Organization of Behavior* (New York: John Wiley & Sons, 1949), 62.

5. D. J. Linden, *The Accidental Mind* (Cambridge: Belknap Press of Harvard University Press, 2007), 42.

6. G. M. Edelman, *Second Nature: Brain Science and Human Knowledge* (New Haven: Yale University Press, 2006), 19.

7. F. Varela, "A Calculus for Self-Reference," *Int. J. General Systems* vol 2. (1975): 5.

8. Varela, "A Calculus," 28.

9. Antonio Damasio, *DesCartes' Error* (New York: G.P. Putnam's Sons, 1994), 143.

10. Damasio, *DesCartes' Error*, 260.

11. Damasio, *DesCartes' Error*, xix.

12. G. Lakoff, and M. Johnson, *Philosophy in the Flesh: The Embodied Mind and Its Challenge to Western Thought* (New York: Basic Books, 1999), 13.

13. Damasio, *DesCartes' Error*, 133.

14. Damasio, *DesCartes' Error*, 139.

15. Damasio, *DesCartes' Error*, 139.

CHAPTER 5: THE BRAIN OF SEX

1. M. Ridley, *The Red Queen: Sex and the Evolution of Human Nature* (New York: Harper Perennial, 2003), 30.

2. Ridley, *The Red Queen*, 30.

3. N. Humphrey, "Conscious Regained: Chapters in the Development of Mind," *A History Of the Mind* (New York: Oxford University Press [VI, rJG], 1983).

4. D. M. Buss, *The Evolution of Desire* (Basic Books, 1994), D. M. Buss et al., "International Preferences in Selecting Mates: A Study of 37 Cultures," *Journal of Cross-Cultural Psychology* 21, no. 1 (1990).

5. L. Brizendine, *The Female Brain* (Morgan Road Books, 2006), 63.

6. D. Morris, *The Human Sexes* (Discovery Channel Video, 1997), D. Morris, *Intimate Behaviour* (New York: Random House, 1971).

7. G. F. Miller, "The Mating Mind: How Sexual Choice Shaped the Evolution of Human Nature," *Psychology* 12 (2001), G. Miller, *The Mating Mind: How Sexual Choice Shaped the Evolution of Human Nature* (New York: Vintage, 2001).

8. "Human Brain Evolution Was a 'Special Event,'" *Howard Hughes Medical News* (December 29, 2004, accessed June 11, 2011. www.hhmi.org/news/lahn3.html).

CHAPTER 6: THE BRAIN OF LOVE AND WAR

1. D. M. Buss, *Evolutionary Psychology: The New Science of the Mind* (New York: Allyn & Bacon, 1999), 31.

2. L. J. Moore, *Sperm Counts: Overcome by Man's Most Precious Fluid* (New York: NYU Press, 2007), 115.

3. G. A. Schuiling, "The Benefit and the Doubt: Why Monogamy?" *J Psychosom Obstet Gynaecol* 24, no. 1 (2003).

4. I. Dupanloup, L. Pereira, G. Bertorelle, F. Calafell, M. J. Prata, A. Amorim, and G. Barbujani, "A Recent Shift from Polygyny to Monogamy in Humans Is Suggested by the Analysis of Worldwide Y-Chromosome Diversity," *Journal of Molecular Evolution* 57, no. 1 (2003).

5. D. Morris, *The Human Sexes: A Natural History of Man and Woman* (New York: Thomas Dunne Books,1998).

6. Buss, *The Evolution of Desire*, 219–20.

7. R. S. McElvaine, *Eve's Seeds: Biology, Sexes, and the Course of History* (New York: McGraw-Hill, 2002), 33.

8. L. H. Keeley, *War Before Civilization* (New York: Oxford University Press US, 1996), 86.

9. N. Wade, *Before the Dawn: Recovering the Lost History of Our Ancestors* (New York: Penguin Press, 2006).

10. M. Twain, *The Adventures of Huckleberry Finn*.

11. N. Wade, "Evolution in History," *Before the Dawn: Recovering the Lost History of Our Ancestors*, (New York: Penguin Press, 2006).

12. Ridley, *The Red Queen: Sex and the Evolution of Human Nature*.

13. Miller, *The Mating Mind: How Sexual Choice Shaped the Evolution of Human Nature*.

14. H. E. Fisher, *Why We Love: The Nature and Chemistry of Romantic Love* (New York: Owl Books, 2005).

15. Brizendine, *The Female Brain*.

16. L. J. Young, "Being Human: Love: NeuroScience Reveals All," *Nature* 457, no. 7226 (2009).

17. Fisher, *Why We Love: The Nature and Chemistry of Romantic Love*.

18. Brizendine, *The Female Brain*.

CHAPTER 7: THE BRAIN OF SONG

1. P. Marler, "Origins of Music and Speech: Insights from Animals," *The Origins of Music* (2000).

2. D. Rothenberg, "Speak Whale to Me," editorial page, *New York Times* (2007).

3. P. J. B. Slater, "Birdsong Repertoires: Their Origins and Use" *The Origins of Music* (2000), 49–63.

4. T. Geissmann, "Gibbon Songs and Human Music from an Evolutionary Perspective." *The Origins of Music* (2000), 103–23.

5. D. A. Schwartz, C. Q. Howe, and D. Purves, "The Statistical Structure of Human Speech Sounds Predicts Musical Universals," *Journal of NeuroScience* 23, no. 18 (2003).

6. S. Kruglinski, *Musical Scales Mimic Sound of Language* (*Discover*, December 2007).

7. Schwartz, Howe, and Purves, "The Statistical Structure of Human Speech Sounds Predicts Musical Universals."

8. S. Brown, "The "Musilanguage" Model of Music Evolution." *The Origins of Music* (2000): 271–300.

9. S. Mithen, I. Morley, A. Wray, M. Tallerman, and C. Gamble, "The Singing Neanderthals," *The Origins of Music, Language, Mind and Body*, by Steven Mithen. (London: Weidenfeld & Nicholson, 2005), 173.

10. Mithen, Morley, Wray, Tallerman, and Gamble, "The Singing Neanderthals," 5.

11. www.wjh.harvard.edu/~mnkylab/media/chimpcalls.html.

12. G. B. Schaller, *The Behavior of the Mountain Gorilla*, 1963.

13. A. C. Arcadi, D. Robert, and C. Boesch, "Buttress Drumming by Wild Chimpanzees: Temporal Patterning, Phrase Integration into Loud Calls, and Preliminary Evidence for Individual Distinctiveness." *Primates* 39, no. 4 (1998): 505–18.

14. J. Goodall, *The Chimpanzees of Gombe: Patterns of Behavior* (Cambridge: Belknap Press of Harvard University Press, 1986).

15. C. Mills, *Boston Globe* on (November 26, 2000), C1.

16. F. B. M. de Waal, "Bonobo Sex and Society," *Scientific American* 272, no. 3 (1995).

17. A. J. Blood, and R. J. Zatorre, "Intensely Pleasurable Responses to Music Correlate with Activity in Brain Regions Implicated in Reward and Emotion," *Proceedings of the National Academy of Sciences* 98, no. 20 (2001).

18. J. A. Seitz, "Dalcroze, "The Body, Movement and Musicality," *Psychology of Music* 33, no. 4 (2005).

19. Choi, "Monkey Drumming Suggests the Origin of Music," *Live Science*, www.liveScience.com/animals/091016-monkey-drumming.html, (2009).

20. C. Darwin, *The Descent of Man, and Selection in Relation to Sex* (1871).

21. G. F. Miller, "Evolution of Human Music through Sexual Selection," (2000).

22. D. Coyle, *The Talent Code* (New York: Bantam Books, 2009).

CHAPTER 8: ETHICS

1. L. W. King, *The Code of Hammurabi*, translated by L. W. King, 1996. Edited by Richard Hooker (1910).

2. J. Rachels and S. Rachels, *The Elements of Moral Philosophy* (Boston: McGraw-Hill, 2007), 143.

3. Rachels and Rachels, *The Elements of Moral Philosophy*,144.

4. Rachels and Rachels, *The Elements of Moral Philosophy*, 132.

5. Rachels and Rachels, *The Elements of Moral Philosophy*, 92.

6. D. Hume, edited by E. F. Miller, *Essays: Moral, Political, and Literary* (Indianapolis: Liberty Classics, 1985), 582.

7. D. Hume, *A Treatise of Human Nature* (Gloucestershire, UK: Clarendon Press, 1888).

8. Hume, *A Treatise of Human Nature*.

9. R. Cohon, "Hume's Moral Philosophy," in *The Stanford Encyclopedia of Philosophy* (2004).

10. L. Arnhart, *Darwinian Natural Right: The Biological Ethics of Human Nature* (Albany: State University of New York Press, 1998), 73.

11. Arnhart, *Darwinian Natural Right*, 73.

12. Darwin, *The Descent of Man, and Selection in Relation to Sex*.

13. Arnhart, *Darwinian Natural Right: The Biological Ethics of Human Nature*.

14. R. Wright, *The Moral Animal: Evolutionary Psychology and Everyday Life* (New York: Vintage Books, 1995),158.

15. M. Ruse, and E. O. Wilson, "Moral Philosophy as Applied Science," *Philosophy*, 61, 236 (1986): 173–92.

16. M. Bekoff, *Wild Justice among Animals*, vol. Sunday, January 25, 2009, Guest Opinions (Boulder, CO: Daily Camera, 2009).

17. M. Bekoff, *The Emotional Lives of Animals: A Leading Scientist Explores Animal Joy, Sorrow, and Empathy—and Why They Matter* (Novato, CA: New World Library, 2007).

18. R. Sapolsky, *Killer Stress*. (Washington, DC: National Geographic, 2003). www.pbs.org/programs/killer-stress/.

19. C. F. Zink et al., "Know Your Place: Neural Processing of Social Hierarchy in Humans," *Neuron* 58, no. 2 (2008).

20. B. Goodman, *Certain Areas of the Brain Size Up Your Competition* (October, 31, 2006 ed., Health: *New York Times*, 2006).

21. N. Angier, *In Pain and Joy of Envy, the Brain May Play a Role*, February, 16, 2009 ed., Science (New York: *New York Times*, 2009).

CHAPTER 9: STORYTELLING AND THE THEORY OF MIND

1. P. C. Hogan, *The Mind and Its Stories: Narrative Universals and Human Emotion*, 3.

2. A. R. Damasio, and H. Damasio, "Brain and Language," *Scientific American* 267, no. 3 (1992).

3. J. Horgan, "Can Science Explain Consciousness?" *Scientific American Book of the Brain*, ed. Editors of Scientific American (Guilford, CN: The Lyons Press, 1999).

4. D. Chalmers, "The Puzzle of Conscious Experience," *Scientific American Book of the Brain*, ed. of *Scientific American* (Guilford, CN: The Lyons Press, 1999).

5. M. S. Gazzaniga, *The Mind's Past* (Berkeley: University of California Press, 2000), J. N. Kotre, *White Gloves: How We Create Ourselves through Memory* (New York: WW Norton & Co., Inc., 1996).

6. G. D. Fireman, O. J. Flanagan, and T. E. McVay. *Narrative and Consciousnes* (Palo Alto, CA: Ebrary), 92.

7. A. Damasio, *Self Comes to Mind* (New York: Pantheon, 2010), 141.

8. Gazzaniga, *The Mind's Past*.

9. J. Bickle, "Empirical Evidence for a Narrative Concept of Self." *Narrative and Consciousness: Literature, Psychology, and the Brain* (2003): 195–208.

10. W. J. Freeman, *Societies of Brains: A Study in the NeuroScience of Love and Hate* (Lawrence Erlbaum, 1995).

11. J. Bering, *The Belief Instinct* (W.W. Norton & Co Inc, 2011), 37.

CHAPTER 10: THE BRAIN OF GOD

1. H. P. Blavatsky, *Thoughts on Ormuzd and Ahriman* (From *Sunrise* magazine, May 1971; copyright © 1971 Theosophical University Press, 1971).

2. A. P. Moller, and R. Thornhill, "Bilateral Symmetry and Sexual Selection: A Meta-Analysis," *The American Naturalist* 151, no. 2 (1998).

3. M. Enquist, and A. Arak, "Symmetry, Beauty, and Evolution," *Nature* 372, no. 6502 (1994).

4. J. R. Rayfield, *The Dualism of Levi-Strauss* (Toronto, Canada: York University, *International Journal of Comparative Sociology*, vol. 12, no. 4, 267–80 (1971), 1971).

5. J. Reynolds, *Jacques Derrida (1930–2004)*, ed. James Fieser, The Internet Encyclopedia of Philosophy (2006).

6. M. Alper, *The "God" Part of the Brain* (New York: Rogue Press, 2001).

7. D. H. Hamer, *The God Gene: How Faith Is Hardwired into Our Genes* (New York: Doubleday, 2004).

8. V. S. Ramachandran, S. Vilayanur, W. S. Hirstein, K. C. Armel, E. Tecoma, and V. Iragul, "The Neural Basis of Religious Experience," (paper presented at the 27th Annual Meeting of the Society for Neuroscience, New Orleans, LA, 1997).

9. M. Shermer, "Why People Believe in God: An Empirical Study on a Deep Question," *The Humanist* (1999).

10. A. B. Newberg, G. D. A. Eugene, and V. Rause, *Why God Won't Go Away: Brain Science and the Biology of Belief* (New York: Ballantine Books, 2001), 26.

11. M. A. Persinger, *Neuropsychological Bases of God Beliefs* (Praeger, 1987).

12. R. Strassman, *DMT: The Spirit Molecule: A Doctor's Revolutionary Research into the Biology of Near-Death and Mystical Experiences* (Park Street Press, 2001), 69.

CHAPTER 11: THE TRICKSTER OF MYTHOLOGY

1. W. J. Hynes, and W. G. Doty, *Mythical Trickster Figures: Contours, Contexts, and Criticisms* (Tuscaloosa: University of Alabama Press, 1993), 226.

2. Hynes and Doty, *Mythical Trickster Figures: Contours, Contexts, and Criticisms*, 34.

3. M. Guenther, *Tricksters and Trancers: Bushman Religion and Society* (Bloomington: Indiana University Press, 1999), 99.

4. Guenther, *Tricksters and Trancers: Bushman Religion and Society*, 97.

5. Encyclopedia Britannica, *Germanic Religion and Mythology*, Germanic-Religion-and-Mythology (2009). www.britannica.com/EBchecked/topic/231102/Germanic-religion-and-mythology/65405/Loki.

6. G. McDermott, *Raven: A Trickster Tale from the Pacific Northwest* (UK; Voyager Books, 2001).

7. Hynes and Doty, *Mythical Trickster Figures: Contours, Contexts, and Criticisms*, 36.

8. P. Radin, K. Kerényi, and C. G. Jung, *The Trickster: A Study in American Indian Mythology* (New York: Schocken Books, 1972).

9. Hynes and Doty, *Mythical Trickster Figures: Contours, Contexts, and Criticisms*.

10. R. D. Pelton, *The Trickster in West Africa: A Study of Mythic Irony and Sacred Delight* (Berkeley: University of California Press, 1989), 36.

11. Pelton, *The Trickster in West Africa: A Study of Mythic Irony and Sacred Delight*, 174.

12. I. Almqvist, *Imelda Almqvist Art: Journeys to Other Worlds, Inner Worlds, and around the World in Paintings*, Paintings of Imelda Almqvist.

13. Hynes and Doty, *Mythical Trickster Figures: Contours, Contexts, and Criticisms*, 35.

14. Hynes and Doty, *Mythical Trickster Figures: Contours, Contexts, and Criticisms*.

15. Radin, Kerényi, and Jung, *The Trickster: A Study in American Indian Mythology*, xxiii.

16. A. Hultkrantz, Professor Emeritus of the Department of Comparative Religion, Stockholm University, *Theories on North American Trickster*, vol. 5, no 2 1997 issue (ACTA AMERICAN, 1997), www.cabiz.net/heartlink/Trickster.htm.

17. F. Boas, *Race, Language, and Culture* (Chicago: University of Chicago Press, 1982), 411.

18. Hultkrantz, *Theories on North American Trickster*.

19. Hultkrantz, *Theories on North American Trickster*.

20. Hynes and Doty, *Mythical Trickster Figures: Contours, Contexts, and Criticisms*.

21. Hynes and Doty, *Mythical Trickster Figures: Contours, Contexts, and Criticisms*.

22. C. Darwin, *The Descent of Man, and Selection in Relation to Sex* (charles-darwin.classic-literature.co.uk/the-descent-of-man/ebook, 1874).

23. Pelton, *The Trickster in West Africa: A Study of Mythic Irony and Sacred Delight*, 255.

24. Hynes and Doty, *Mythical Trickster Figures: Contours, Contexts, and Criticisms*.

CHAPTER 12: A SWATH OF TRICKSTER STORIES FROM ORAL LITERATURE

1. F. Ballinger, "Living Sideways: Social Themes and Social Relationships in Native American Trickster Tales," *American Indian Quarterly* 13, no. 1 (1989).

2. B. H. Lopez, "Coyote Marries a Man" *Giving Birth to Thunder, Sleeping with His Daughter: Coyote Builds North America* (Harper Perennial, 1990), 61.

3. R. Benedict, "Coyote and Beaver Exchange Wives," *Tales of the Cochiti Indians* (Forgotten Books 2008), 186.

4. R. Erdoes, and A. Ortiz, "The Winkte Way," *American Indian Trickster Tales* (University of Nebraska Press, 1987).

5. R. D. Pelton, *The Trickster in West Africa: A Study of Mythic Irony and Sacred Delight* (University of California Press, 1989), 36.

6. B. H. Lopez, "Coyote Visits the Women" *Giving Birth to Thunder, Sleeping with His Daughter: Coyote Builds North America by Barry H. Lopez* (Harper Perennial, 1990), 148.

7. B. H. Lopez, "Coyote and His Anus" *Giving Birth to Thunder, Sleeping with His Daughter: Coyote Builds North America* by Barry H. Lopez (Harper Perennial, 1990).

8. P. Radin, *The Trickster* (Schocken 1987).

9. R. Dorie, *Tales of Uncle Tompa* (Barrytown/Station Hill Press, Inc., 1997).

10. C. H. Berndt, and Ronald M. Berndt, *The World of the First Australians: Aboriginal Traditional Life: Past and Present* (Aboriginal Studies Press, 1988).

11. R. Erdoes, and A. Ortiz, "Coyote Sleeps with His Own Daughters," *American Indian Trickster Tales* (University of Nebraska Press, 1987).

12. H. Scheub, "How Kwaku Ananse Got Aso in Marriage," *African Tales* (The University of Wisconsin Press, 2005 by the Board of Regents of the University of Wisconsin System. Reprinted by permission of The University of Wisconsin), 3–7.

13. R. Erdoes, and A. Ortiz, "Coyote Keeps His Dead Wife's Genitals," *American Indian Trickster Tales* (University of Nebraska Press, 1987).

CHAPTER 13: FEMALE TRICKSTERS

1. H. L. Gates, *The Signifying Monkey: A Theory of African-American Literary Criticism* (New York: Oxford University Press, 1989), 29.

2. M. Jurich, *Scheherazade's Sisters: Trickster Heroines and Their Stories in World Literature* (Greenwood Press, 1998), 2.

3. Jurich, *Scheherazade's Sisters*, 3.

4. F. Ballinger, "Coyote, He/She Was Going There: Sex and Gender in Native American Trickster Stories," *Studies in American Indian Literatures: The Journal of the Association for the Study of American Indian Literatures* 12, no. 4 (2000).

5. L. Landay, *Madcaps, Screwballs, and Con Women: Female Trickster in American Culture* (Philadelphia: University of Pennsylvania Press, 1998), 2.

6. R. Erdoes, and A. Oriz, "The Toothed Vagina," *American Indian Trickster Tales* (New York: Viking/Penguin, 1998).

7. R. Erdoes, and A. Oriz, "Teeth in the Wrong Place," *American Indian Trickster Tales* (New York: Viking/Penguin, 1998).

8. R. Erdoes, and A. Oriz, "Old Coyote Woman Meets Old Coyote Man," *American Indian Trickster Tales* (New York: Viking/Penguin, 1998).

9. A. S. Rappoport, "The Most Precious Thing in the World," *The Folklore of the Jews*: (Bel Air, CA: Singing Tree Press, 1972).

10. A. K. Ramanujan, "The Wife Who Refused to Be Beaten," *Folktales From India* (New York: Pantheon, 1994).

CHAPTER 14: LITERARY FILTERS

1. T. Eagleton, *Literary Theory: An Introduction* (University of Minnesota Press), 116.

2. P. Gowaty, *Feminism and Evolutionary Biology: Boundaries, Intersections, and Frontiers* (Springer, 1997), 23.

3. Gowaty, *Feminism and Evolutionary Biology*, 25.

4. Gowaty, *Feminism and Evolutionary Biology*, 27.

5. Gowaty, *Feminism and Evolutionary Biology*, 25.

6. Gowaty, *Feminism and Evolutionary Biology*, 29.

7. M. Ridley, *The Red Queen: Sex and the Evolution of Human Nature* (Perennial, 2003), 261.

CHAPTER 15: MUSIC AND THE TRICKSTER

1. M. K. Asante, and A. S. Abarry, *African Intellectual Heritage: A Book of Sources* (Philadelphia: Temple University Press, 1996), xiii.

2. A. Ruoff, "Lavonne Brown," *American Indian Literatures: An Introduction, Bibliographic Review, and Selected Bibliography*.

3. *"Apache Creation Story"* (www.indians.org/welker/creation.htm).

4. E. W. Reed, "Bunjil the Creator," *Aboriginal Myths and Legends* (New Holland Australia,1999).

5. "Diné (or Navajo) Creation Story" (www-bcf.usc.edu/~lapahie/Creation. html).

6. Oyekan Owomoyela, *Yoruba Trickster Tales* (University of Nebraska Press,1997), xiii.

7. R. Erdoes, and A. Ortiz, "Coyote Giving," *American Indian Trickster Tales* (Viking/Penguin, 1998).

8. R. Leadbetter, *Hermes* (Encyclopedia Mythica, www.pantheon.org/articles/h/hermes.html, 2006).

9. K. C. Aryan, *Hanuman: Art, Mythology & Folklore* (New Dehli: B. Nath, 1994).

10. Aryan, *Hanuman.*

11. Aryan, *Hanuman.*

12. E. E. Evans-Pritchard, *The Zande Trickster* (Cambridge: Published by Oxford, Clarendon P, 1967), 90.

CHAPTER 16: A SWATH OF OTHER TRICKSTER STORIES FROM AROUND THE WORLD

1. J. C. Harris, "The Wonderful Tar Baby Story," *Uncle Remus and Legends of the Old Plantation* (www.en.utexas.edu/amlit/amlitprivate/texts/remus.htm).

2. A. Lang, "How the Wicked Tanuki Was Punished," *The Crimson Fairy Book* (www.classicreader.com/book/971/29).

3. J. Bierhorst, *Latin American Folktales: Stories from Hispanic and Indian Traditions* (Pantheon),195.

4. A. C. Yu, *Journey to the West*, vol. 1 (University Of Chicago Press, 1980), 103.

5. "The Wanderings of Dionysus" (www.sacred-texts.com/etc/omw/omw35.htm).

6. "Orphesus" (www.sacred-texts.com/etc/omw/omw34.htm).

7. T. Burke, ed. *De infantia Iesu euangelium Thomae graece, Corpus Christianorum Series Apocryphorum* vol. 17 (Turnhout, Brepols, 2011).

8. J. Bierhorst, *Latin American Folktales: Stories from Hispanic and Indian Traditions* (Pantheon), 213.

9. *We-gyet: Legends of the Northwest.* (Hancock Wildlife Foundation, 2006).

CHAPTER 17: THE TRICKSTER PERSONIFIED

1. J. Tierney, *Why We Laugh*, HealthScience (*New York Times*, 2007).

2. Tierney, *Why We Laugh.*

3. P. D. McClean, *Brain Evolution Relating to Family, Play, and the Separation Call.* (Arch Gen Psychiatry. 1985 April 42[4]:405–17, 1985).

4. J. Fire, and R. Erdoes, *Lame Deer: Seeker of Visions* (A Touchstone Book, 1972), 249.

5. S. Mizrach, *Thunderbird and Trickster*, ed. Dr. Steven Mizrach, Cyber Anthropology, www.fiu.edu/~Mizrachs/Cyberanthropos.html.

6. J. H. Steward, "The Clown in Native North America," (Berkeley: University of California, Berkeley, 1929).

7. Steward, "The Clown in Native North America."

8. Steward, "The Clown in Native North America."

9. Steward, "The Clown in Native North America."

10. Steward, "The Clown in Native North America."

11. Steward, "The Clown in Native North America."

12. Steward, "The Clown in Native North America."

13. Steward, "The Clown in Native North America."

14. Red Elk, *Sacred Fools and Clowns* (www.redelk.net/website/heyoka.htm).

15. R. J. DeMallie, *The Sixth Grandfather: Black Elk's Teachings Given to John G. Neihardt* (Lincoln: University of Nebraska Press, 1985), 232–35.

16. K. Dowman, translator, *The Divine Madman: The Sublime Life and Songs of Krukpa Kunley: A Compilation of Anecdotes and Songs Complied by the Bhutanese Scholar, Geshe Chaphu, in 1966* (London: Rider & Co, 1982), 95–98.

17. S. Goodman, *Wisdom Crazy: An Interview with Steven Goodman*, Inquiring Mind (www.inquiringmind.com/Articles/WisdomCrazy.html, 2005).

18. W. Nisker, *The Essential Crazy Wisdom* (Berkeley, CA: Ten Speed Press, 1990).

19. S. Goodman, *Wisdom Crazy: An Interview with Steven Goodman*, Inquiring Mind (www.inquiringmind.com/Articles/WisdomCrazy.html, 2005).

20. L. Stryk, *The Penguin Book of Zen Poetry* (Athens: Ohio University Press, 1978), 16.

21. L. Stryk, *The Penguin Book of Zen Poetry* (Athens: Ohio University Press, 1978), 16.

22. D. L. Puji, *Wudeng Huiyan* (Compendium of Five Lamps). Translated by Andy Ferguson (Boston: Wisdom Publications, 2000).

23. P. N. Gregory, *Sudden and Gradual: Approaches to Enlightenment in Chinese Thought* (Motilal Books, January 1, 1991), 419.

24. W. Whitman, *Leaves of Grass* (New York: Oxford University Press, 2005), 48.

25. K. Yamada, *The Gateless Gate: The Classic Book of Zen Koans* (Wisdom Publications, 2004), 69.

26. L. Stryk, *The Penguin Book of Zen Poetry* (Athens: Ohio University Press, 1978), 16.

27. Patterson and Robinsin, translators. *The Nag Hammadi Library*. (www.gnosis.org/naghamm/gth_pat_rob.htm).

28. E. A. Stewart, *Jesus the Holy Fool* (Sheed & Ward, 1999), 114.

29. M. G. Guenther, *Tricksters and Trancers: Bushman Religion and Society* (Bloomington: Indiana University Press, 1999), 181.

30. J. M. Kats, *Het Javaansch Tooneel—Wajong Poerwa*, Weltevreden; Volks-Lectuur (1923), J. L. Peacock, "Symbolic Reversal and Social History:

Transvestites and Clowns of Java," *The Reversible World: Symbolic Inversion in Art and Society* [*Papers*] (1972).

31. W. Nisker, *The Essential Crazy Wisdom* (Berkeley, CA: Ten Speed Press, 1990), 50.

32. M. Bakhtin, *Rabelais and His World* (Bloomington: Indiana University Press, 1984), 50.

33. B. K. Otto, *Fools Are Everywhere: The Court Jester around the World* (Chicago: University of Chicago Press, 2001)

34. Otto, *Fools Are Everywhere*, 32.

35. Otto, *Fools Are Everywhere*, 32.

36. Otto, *Fools Are Everywhere*, 32.

37. Otto, *Fools Are Everywhere*, 32.

38. E. Welsford, *The Fool: His Social and Literary History* (Faber and Faber, 1935), 93.

39. Welsford, *The Fool*, 32.

40. A. K. Ramanujan, "How Tali Rama Became a Jester," *Folktales from India* (Pantheon Fairy Tale & Folklore Library, 1991).

41. J. Yolen, "Tyll Ulenspiegel's Merry Prank" *Favorite Folktales from Around the World, Pantheon Fairy Tale and Folklore Library* (Pantheon1988), 128.

42. J. Yolen, "Quevedo and the King" *Favorite Folktales from Around the World, Pantheon Fairy Tale and Folklore Library* (Pantheon1988), 131.

CHAPTER 18: BLUES AND COURTING TRICKSTERS

1. B. Robertson, *Little Blues Book* (Algonquin Books of Chapel Hill, 1996).

2. A. Y. Davis, *Blues Legacies and Black Feminism: Gertrude" Ma" Rainey, Bessie Smith, and Billie Holiday* (Pantheon Books, 1998), 10.

3. F. Ballinger, "Living Sideways: Social Themes and Social Relationships in Native American Trickster Tales," *American Indian Quarterly* (1989), 56.

4. W. T. Lhamon, *Raising Cain: Blackface Performance from Jim Crow to Hip Hop* (Harvard University Press, 1998), 24.

5. G. Oakley, *The Devil's Music: A History of the Blues* (Da Capo Pr, 1997), 91.

6. A. Y. Davis, *Blues Legacies and Black Feminism: Gertrude" Ma" Rainey, Bessie Smith, and Billie Holiday* (Pantheon Books, 1998), 214.

7. Davis, *Blues Legacies and Black Feminism*, 238.

8. Davis, *Blues Legacies and Black Feminism*, 9.

9. J. R. Desmond, *Bessie Smith 1894-1937*, The Tennessee Encyclopedia of History and Culture (Tennessee Historical Society, Nashville, Tennesseee, tennesseeencyclopedia.net/imagegallery.php?EntryID=S045, 1998).

10. Davis, *Blues Legacies and Black Feminism*, 328.

11. Jefferson, Blind Lemon, "Black Snake Moan" (www.lyricstime.com/blind-lemon-jefferson-that-black-snake-moan-lyrics.html).

12. G. Oakley, *The Devil's Music: A History Of The Blues* (1st De Capo Pres, 1983), 55.

13. F. Davis, *The History of the Blues*, (Mojo Working Productions),106.

14. Davis, *The History of the Blues*, 106.

15. E. Wald, *Escaping the Delta: Robert Johnson and the Invention of the Blues* (Amistad, 2004).

16. Wald, *Escaping the Delta*, 275.

17. McKinley (Muddy Waters) Morganfield, "Nineteen Years Old" (blueslyrics.tripod.com/lyrics/muddy_waters/she_s_nineteen_years_old.htm).

18. B. Tindall. *Mozart in the Jungle* (New York: Atlantic Monthly Press, 2005), 96.

CHAPTER 19: TRICKSTER IN WRITTEN LITERATURE

1. A. Bilger, *Laughing Feminism: Subversive Comedy in Frances Burney, Maria Edgeworth, and Jane Austen* (Detroit: Wayne State University Press, 1998), 89.

2. D. J. Williams, *"Laughing Lion, and Shadows"* (unpublished essay, 2007).

3. B. A. Babcock, *The Reversible World: Symbolic Inversion in Art and Society* (Ithaca: Cornell University Press, 1978).

4. G. Chaucer, L. D. Benson translator, *The Canterbury Tales Complete* (New York: Wadsworth Publishing, 2000).

5. M. M. Bakhtin, M. Holquist, and C. Emerson, *The Dialogic Imagination: Four Essays* (Austin: University of Texas Press, 1981), 273.

CHAPTER 20: TRICKSTER WAS WANDERING

1. J. Fire and R. Erdoes, *Lame Deer: Seeker of Visions* (A Touchstone Book, 1972), 75.

2. E. H. Pagels, *Adam, Eve and the Serpent* (Random House, 1988), 145.

INDEX

ABOUT THE AUTHOR

David Williams has been working in the arts all of his life, as a writer, musician, singer-songwriter, and cartoonist (including a long-time stint with *The Chronicle of Higher Education*). In 2009 he won an Emmy for his work as a songwriter for a PBS children's show, and two of his books for children were published by Alfred A. Knopf. He has published a book of short stories with Ghost Road Press, *Indian Bingo*, with a corresponding collection of songs that mirror the characters in the book, *Joplin, MO*. David's latest CD for adults, *Chocolate Bar,* a collection of original americana music, hit the Top 40 in the US and European americana charts in 2011. Videos of his songs on YouTube from the PBS show have had over thirty million hits.

David has been a writer-in-residence at a number of universities and colleges, including Knox College and the Metropolitan State College of Denver. Currently, he teaches in the Writing Program at CU, Boulder. He has a PhD in English is from the University of Illinois at Chicago, a MA in English from Northern Illinois University, and a BA in anthropology from Northern Illinois University.

Ingram Content Group UK Ltd.
Milton Keynes UK
UKHW041619070323
418181UK00002B/16

9 780739 143971